Presented
with the compliments of
Geigy Pharmaceuticals

Paediatric Perspectives
on Epilepsy

Paediatric Perspectives on Epilepsy

Symposium held at the
Grand Hotel, Eastbourne,
December 1984

Edited by

EUAN ROSS
Charing Cross Hospital, London, UK

and

EDWARD REYNOLDS
King's College Hospital, London, UK

A Wiley Medical Publication

JOHN WILEY & SONS
Chichester · New York · Brisbane · Toronto · Singapore

Library of Congress Cataloging in Publication Data:
Main entry under title:

Paediatric perspectives on epilepsy.
   (A Wiley medical publication)
   Includes index.
   1. Epilepsy in children—Congresses. I. Ross,
Euan M. II. Reynolds, Edward. III. Series. [DNLM: 1. Epilepsy—in infancy &
childhood—congresses. WL 385 P123 1984]
RJ496.E6P34 1985   618.92'853   85-12009

ISBN 0 471 90817 7

British Library Cataloguing in Publication Data:

Paediatric perspectives on epilepsy:
   Symposium held at the Grand Hotel, Eastbourne,
   December 1984.
   1.   Epilepsy in children
   I.   Ross, Euan II. Reynolds, Edward
618.92'853   RJ496.E6

ISBN 0 471 90817 7

Phototypeset by Dobbie Typesetting Service, Plymouth, Devon
Printed and bound in Great Britain

Contents

Part III: Epilepsy in the pre-school child

Part IV: The schoolchild

Chairmen and Contributors

Douglas Addy, *Dudley Road Hospital, Birmingham*

Jean Aicardi, *Hôpital des Enfants Malades, Paris*

Martin Bellman, *Royal National Throat, Nose and Ear Hospital, London*

Keith Brown, *Royal Hospital for Sick Children, Edinburgh*

John Corbett, *Bethlem Royal Hospital, London*

Orvar Eeg-Olofsson, *University Hospital, Linköping, Sweden*

Stuart Green, *Institute of Child Health, Birmingham*

Gwilym Hosking, *Children's Hospital, Sheffield*

Malcolm Levene, *Royal Infirmary, Leicester*

John Livingston, *Royal Hospital for Sick Children, Edinburgh*

Breege MacArdle, *King's College Hospital, London*

Ian McKinlay, *Booth Hall Children's Hospital, Manchester*

Brian Neville, *Guy's Hospital, London*

Niall O'Donohoe, *National Children's Hospital, Dublin*

Leon Polnay, *Queen's Medical Centre, University of Nottingham*

Edward Reynolds, *King's College Hospital, London*

Richard Robinson, *Guy's Hospital, London*

Euan Ross, *Charing Cross Hospital, London*

Pamela Thompson, *National Hospitals for Nervous Diseases, London*

Michael Trimble, *National Hospitals for Nervous Diseases, London*

Christopher Verity, *Bristol Royal Hospital for Sick Children, Bristol*

Organizing Committee

David Lott
Edward Reynolds
Euan Ross
Michael Trimble

Preface

Among the problems that confound clinicians who care for children, epilepsy in its many paediatric forms ranks high as an area where good practice yields much benefit to the affected child – and great harm can be done by the uninformed. Overmedication is often more harmful than the converse, and all too often children are needlessly labelled 'epileptic'. To the non-specialist, epilepsies in childhood may seem a somewhat static bywater of medicine; to the initiated this is very far from the case. Children's epilepsy is now attracting high-calibre research-minded clinicians and specialists in basic sciences. As a result some of its mysteries are starting to crack under the onslaught of intensive epidemiological, immunological and neuro-investigatory studies. Unfortunately, this new knowledge is taking a long time to reach the standard medical textbooks and hence filter into clinical practice.

In order to speed up this process, a conference was held at the end of 1984 where clinicians active in research into children's epilepsy were invited to share their knowledge with a large audience of younger paediatricians and other clinicians. In this book we publish their texts, spiced with highlights from the formal discussion. Although we could not capture in print the extended and often passionate discussions that went on outside the conference chamber, we hope that we have captured something of the state of the art of practical care of the child with epilepsy – in this, the first European multi-authored book on children's epilepsy.

EUAN ROSS

Acknowledgements

Dr George Birdwood undertook the detailed preparation of this book, and the volume editor and publishers would like to express their gratitude for his enthusiastic hard work.

Part I: Seizures in the newborn

Paediatric Perspectives on Epilepsy
Edited by E. Ross and E. Reynolds
© 1985 John Wiley & Sons Ltd.

1

Causation of seizures

NIALL O'DONOHOE
Department of Paediatrics, National Children's Hospital, Dublin

SUMMARY

Every patient with suspected epilepsy calls for a correct diagnosis, which should include both a seizure diagnosis and an aetiological diagnosis. The current concept of the aetiology of the epilepsies is that they are multifactorial in causation, with genetic and acquired factors operating to varying degrees in each case. Most human epilepsies, whether generalized or partial, appear to share a common genetic basis which contributes significantly to epileptogenesis. In childhood, the different types of seizure characteristic of certain age groups reflect the stage of maturation of the developing brain. Although the interaction between exogenous factors and inherited predisposition is not understood, it seems likely that the process of kindling plays an important role. In addition, the actual occurrence of seizures appears to predispose an individual to further seizures. Biological trigger factors precipitate many seizures, particularly in early childhood.

INTRODUCTION

Seizures are among the most frequent symptoms in paediatrics and constitute the commonest symptom of all those presenting to the paediatric neurologist. More than 75% of patients with epilepsy begin having their seizures before 18 years of age. This must be related to the propensity of the developing nervous system to produce seizure discharges – which can be documented both clinically and experimentally.

The cause of epilepsy has been a subject of speculation since earliest times. Hippocrates attributed it to natural biological causes, primarily heredity. Hughlings Jackson (1873) wrote that: 'epilepsy is the name of occasional, sudden, excessive, rapid and local discharges of grey matter'. The EEG,

3

discovered subsequently by Hans Berger, provided visual evidence for the truth of this statement. We now know that the paroxysmal depolarization shift is the long-lasting alteration in potential which occurs in damaged neurones and leads to the bursting pattern of firing which is their hallmark. Pools of damaged neurones firing together produce the characteristic EEG spike.

DIAGNOSIS AND CLASSIFICATION

Epilepsy presents clinically as a paroxysmal disorder with recurring seizures as its symptoms. The seizures may be experienced subjectively, described by a witness, or photographed and analysed by camera and EEG. History, physical examination, laboratory studies, EEG, computer tomography (CT) and other sophisticated techniques enable us to diagnose epilepsy much more precisely than in the past, and to study its nature.

The three main tasks facing us when a child or adult presents with epilepsy are: (1) making a correct diagnosis; (2) identifying the seizure type; and (3) attempting to establish a cause. We need to make both a *seizure diagnosis* to identify the seizure type, and an *aetiological diagnosis* to identify the cause of the seizures. The search for both diagnoses is necessary for the proper care of the patient with epilepsy.

Seizures may broadly be divided into: (a) *generalized seizures*, which are bilaterally symmetrical and without local onset; and (b) *partial seizures*, with a local onset, which may become secondarily generalized. Some writers on epilepsy have had doubts about the wisdom of regarding seizures as symptoms. Lennox (1960) felt that regarding epilepsy solely as a symptom led to defeatism about the search for causes. He proposed that: 'as a brain disorder epilepsy is a disease but as a seizure it is a symptom.' Seizures are evidence of a sick or malfunctioning brain.

When does a series of symptoms become a disease entity? When a common cause can be found. The triad of fever, cough and weight loss was called 'consumption' until Koch identified the tubercle bacillus. In the case of epilepsy, the question of a disease entity is obscured because seizures may result from virtually all the serious diseases of humankind: congenital malformations, infections, vascular diseases, tumours, trauma, degenerative diseases. So the problem of aetiology is scattered into a hundred parts, a hundred epilepsies or epileptic syndromes.

AETIOLOGY

Four positions are possible with regard to aetiology:

(1) *All epilepsies are primary/essential/functional, and brain lesions, even if present, are without influence.* This is untenable because we know, for example, that trauma and tumour can lead to epilepsy.

(2) *All epilepsies are secondary/symptomatic/lesional.* As a symptom the seizure is then like a headache – with a multitude of causes but no common cause. All causes would be acquired and no epilepsy inherited except as a symptom of a congenital brain defect.

(3) *Primary and secondary epilepsies exist but are mutually exclusive.* Seizures may come either out of a clear sky or out of a sky clouded by brain insult.

(4) *Primary and secondary epilepsies are not mutually exclusive,* and the factor common to all persons subject to seizures is the diathesis, the predisposition, the susceptibility to seizures, the 'epileptogenicity' of the individual.

The fourth possibility is the only tenable one for most cases, although examples of the first two possibilities exist where genetically-determined epileptogenicity is either maximal or minimal.

Lennox (1960) compared diathesis to a combustible material of greater or lesser inflammability, which differs in the facility with which it will ignite but which will unfailingly do so if a flame of sufficient intensity is applied. The first possibility represents spontaneous combustion, whereas the second (i.e. entirely secondary epilepsies) represents relatively incombustible material being set alight by the flame of convulsant drugs or severe brain damage. The current concept of the aetiology of the epilepsies is that they are multifactorial in causation with genetic and acquired factors operating to varying degrees in each case.

MODES OF INHERITANCE . . .

More than 100 single-gene disorders may be associated with epilepsy, including autosomal dominant conditions like tuberous sclerosis, recessive conditions such as Tay–Sachs disease, and X-linked conditions such as Menkes's syndrome. With the addition of chromosomal disorders which are associated with epilepsy, such as trisomy 13 and 18, these account for less than 2% of all childhood epilepsies.

Metrakos and Metrakos (1961), in a classic study, took probands with absence attacks and/or major generalized grand mal, no obvious neuropathology, and paroxysmal bilaterally synchronous 3 Hz spike-wave EEG discharges. From studies of the relatives, they postulated that the spike-wave trait, not the epilepsy, was inherited, and that it was inherited as an autosomal dominant with age-dependent penetrance. Penetrance was very low at birth, rose rapidly to nearly complete penetrance (i.e. expression in almost 50% of first-degree relatives) around 10 years of age and then declined gradually to almost no penetrance at 40 years.

The prevalence of the 3 Hz spike-wave trait was found to be almost as high in the relatives of probands with one or more febrile seizures, another condition with a strong genetic predisposition.

The siblings and offspring of patients with petit mal absences and 3 Hz spike-wave EEG discharges were found to have:

(a)   a 50% risk of inheriting the gene for the spike-wave EEG abnormality;
(b)   a 35% risk of expressing that EEG trait at any time;
(c)   a 12% risk of having one or two seizures;
(d)   an 8% risk of developing primary generalized seizures.

This last category represents a low risk, much below that of recessive or dominant inheritance (25% or 50%).

. . . AND INTERACTION

Partial or focal epilepsies have long been attributed to environmental causes. Andermann (1980) in Montreal has analysed the aetiological factors in 60 patients operated on for focal epilepsy and found *perinatal factors*, *infections* and *postnatal trauma* to be the most significant, in that order. Studying their families, she found no significant increase in seizures in first-, second- and third-degree relatives, compared with controls, but there was a significant increase in EEG abnormalities, including those associated with epilepsy. It is postulated that, in focal epilepsy, a number of exogenous variables must interact with the genotype in order to produce the final clinical and EEG phenotype for epilepsy.

In spite of the multiplicity of exogenous factors which can cause recurrent epileptic seizures, most human epilepsies, whether generalized or partial, share a common genetic basis which significantly contributes to epileptogenesis. This genetically-determined potentially epileptogenic brain dysfunction reveals itself in the EEG by generalized spike-wave discharges (Gloor, 1982). These are the neurophysiological expression of a diffuse corticoreticular hyperexcitability, brought about, at cellular level, by biochemical abnormalities – possibly including the abnormal leakage of glutamic acid into the extracellular compartment. Inherited epileptogenicity must interact with other aetiological factors, some of them probably also genetic but the majority exogenous, encompassing the long list of pathological states recognized as causing epilepsy. These exogenous factors by themselves are not capable of causing epilepsy, but must interact with the genetic predisposition to corticoreticular hyperexcitability to do so. As Doose (1980) expresses it, organic brain lesions may represent what he calls a 'realisation factor' for clinical expression of the epileptic phenotype. In an apparently primary epilepsy, a trivial brain insult may bring the epilepsy to clinical expression; contrariwise, among children with epilepsy manifesting itself exclusively on a basis of brain damage, Doose found additional genetic factors in 70%.

KINDLING

We do not know how this interaction works – why a genetic predisposition becomes clinically manifest in one child while a sibling with the same predisposition remains healthy. The explanation may reside in the factor we call *kindling*, defined as 'igniting and spreading like fire', that is used to describe a process in which regular repetition of a stimulus in the brain leads to a permanent augmentation of response. An initially subconvulsive intracerebral electrical stimulus is repeated and eventually causes a convulsive response each time it is applied.

Many consider kindling to be the key phenomenon in the pathophysiology of epilepsy (Glaser, 1983). The basis for it is unknown. Does kindling, over a period of time, produce morphological changes in neurones, their dendrites, axons and vesicles containing neurotransmitters, leading to the altered transmission of impulses and, sometimes, the development of secondary or 'mirror' foci? It has been shown, in primates, that an animal genetically predisposed to seizures can be kindled faster than an apparently non-epileptic animal. Is this a model for the interaction of an acquired lesion with epileptogenicity in the human?

Kindling has been demonstrated in different parts of the brain but especially in the limbic areas. We are reminded of the scarring produced by a prolonged febrile convulsion in infancy, leading to the interactable complex partial seizures of temporal lobe epilepsy later. Trimble (1981) has suggested that the kindling phenomenon may not be limited to seizures, but may also be responsible for inducing behavioural and psychiatric disorders with temporal lobe seizures by means of persisting electrical activity in the limbic circuits.

THE GOWERS PHENOMENON

Reynolds (1981) has referred more than once in his writings to what he calls 'the Gowers phenomenon', quoting Gowers (1881):

> 'The effect of a convulsion on the nerve centres is such as to render the occurrence of another more easy, to intensify the predisposition that already exists. Thus every fit may be said to be, in part, the result of those which have preceded it, the cause of those which follow it.'

This is clearly an argument for the early and active treatment of epilepsy, as Shorvon and Reynolds (1982) have demonstrated in adults.

TRIGGER FACTORS

We should not forget the role of biological changes as triggering factors in the causation of clinical seizures: for example, fever, infection, emotional upset, excessive fatigue, lack of sleep, overhydration and alcohol, biochemical changes such as hypoglycaemia, hypocalcaemia and the results of hypernatraemia and, of course, the precipitate withdrawal of drugs.

THE OVERALL PICTURE

The factors we have considered in the causation of epilepsy include heredity, structural brain disease, age and biological changes. Similarly, Lennox (1960) stated that: 'The type of epilepsy which occurs in a child represents a confluence of age, heredity, and structural brain abnormality.'

Taking all these matters about aetiology into account, one may attempt to classify the epilepsies or epileptic syndromes into two main groups, as either:

(a) *Primary* or *essential* or *functional* or *genetic* epilepsies, independent of an identifiable brain lesion; or
(b) *Secondary* or *symptomatic* or *lesional* epilepsies, dependent on the presence of a brain lesion.

From what has been said already, it should be clear that this is an oversimplification of the problem. The main difference between primary and secondary epilepsies lies in the special weight of the different genetic and exogenous factors in each individual epilepsy. The difference between the two groups is, accordingly, more relative than absolute. Nevertheless, the division remains a useful one in practice and is especially relevant in relation to prognosis.

Primary epilepsies are dependent on a constitutional predisposition characterized by a lower seizure threshold. The onset of a specific type of seizure at a specific age distinguishes the primary epilepsies. Many of them, both generalized and partial, run a self-limited course and eventually go into complete and permanent remission. It has been estimated that one in four children with epilepsy may have a benign form. This concept of benign or self-limited epilepsy has evolved in the past 25 years and includes both generalized and partial epilepsies. Characteristically, in benign epilepsy: (a) there is no associated neurological deficit; (b) the seizures are mild and usually infrequent; (c) the response to therapy is usually satisfactory (and some patients do not require therapy); and (d) the prognosis is excellent with or without treatment.

The best-known of these benign epileptic syndromes is probably the benign focal epilepsy of childhood, also called Rolandic, Sylvian or benign centro-temporal epilepsy, which is now recognized as one of the most frequent forms of epilepsy in childhood, accounting for 15% or more. In all of these epilepsies one may expect to find evidence of inherited epileptogenicity strongly represented.

CONCLUSION

Epilepsy is not the great unknown, nor the mystery disease, nor an idiopathic or cryptogenic condition, nor a 'disease of undetermined aetiology'. Regarding it as such does a disservice to ourselves, to the scientific basis of medicine and to our patients. Understanding its aetiology helps us to learn more about it and to treat it more effectively.

REFERENCES

ANDERMANN, E. (1980) Multifactorial inheritance in the epilepsies. In: *Advances in Epileptology. The XIth Epilepsy International Symposium*, pp. 297–310 (Eds R. Canger, F. Angeleri, and J. K. Penry). Raven Press, New York.

DOOSE, H. (1980) Genetic factors in childhood epilepsy. In: *Advances in Epileptology. The XIth Epilepsy International Symposium*, pp. 289–296 (Eds R. Canger, F. Angeleri, and J. K. Penry). Raven Press, New York.

GLASER, G. H. (1983) Kindling. *Dev. Med. Child Neurol.*, **25**, 376–380.

GLOOR, P. (1982) Toward a unifying concept of epileptogenesis. In: *Advances in Epileptology. The XIIIth Epilepsy International Symposium*, p. 86 (Eds H. Akimoto, H. Kazamatsuri, M. Seino *et al.*). Raven Press, New York.

GOWERS, W. R. (1881) *Epilepsy and Other Chronic Convulsive Disorders: Their Causes, Symptoms and Treatment*. Churchill, London.

JACKSON, J. HUGHLINGS (1931–32) *Selected Writings of John Hughlings Jackson*, p. 100 (Ed. J. Taylor). Hodder and Stoughton, London.

LENNOX, W. G. (Ed.) (1960) Areas of orientation. In: *Epilepsy and Related Disorders*, Vol. I, pp. 51–56. Churchill, London.

METRAKOS, K., and METRAKOS, J. D. (1961) Genetics of convulsive disorders. II. Genetic and electroencephalographic studies in centrencephalic epilepsy. *Neurology*, **2**, 474–483.

REYNOLDS, E. H. (1981) Biological factors in psychological disorders associated with epilepsy. In: *Epilepsy and Psychiatry*, pp. 264–290 (Eds E. H. Reynolds and M. R. Trimble). Churchill Livingstone, Edinburgh.

SHORVON, S. D., and REYNOLDS, E. H. (1982) Early prognosis of epilepsy. *Br. Med. J.*, **285**, 1699–1701.

TRIMBLE, M. R. (1981) The limbic system. In: *Epilepsy and Psychiatry*, pp. 216–226 (Eds E. H. Reynolds and M. R. Trimble). Churchill Livingstone, Edinburgh.

Paediatric Perspectives on Epilepsy
Edited by E. Ross and E. Reynolds
© 1985 John Wiley & Sons Ltd.

2

Aetiology of neonatal seizures

MALCOLM I. LEVENE
Neonatal Unit, Department of Child Health, Leicester University Medical School

SUMMARY

There is a wide range of causes for neonatal convulsions, but in published reports idiopathic seizures are found in up to one-third of all cases. In 46 full-term infants admitted with seizures to the Leicester Royal Infirmary during the first month of life, a definite diagnosis was reached in all but two cases. Asphyxia remained the commonest single cause (52% of cases). Haemorrhage was demonstrated by real-time ultrasound in eight (17%) – four intraventricular, one primary intracerebral, two thalamic, and one subarachnoid. Three infants with fits were found to have sustained cerebral artery infarction. Without ultrasound scanning, these 11 cases would probably have been described as idiopathic. Other causes included: *infection* in seven, *hypoglycaemia* in four, and *metabolic disorders* in seven. Meningo-encephalitis, developmental abnormalities of the brain and the effects of narcotic withdrawal can also cause neonatal seizures. The incidence of seizures in the newborn has been increasing over the last decade, probably as a result of increasingly frequent referral for investigation. Imaging techniques as well as continuous EEG monitoring may well improve diagnostic accuracy in neonatal seizures and more often elucidate their cause.

INTRODUCTION

The frequency of convulsions depends on the diagnostic criteria used to define seizures, the gestational age of the infant and the population of neonates from which the sample is drawn. The incidence of neonatal convulsions in infants admitted to the Special Care Baby Unit of a district general hospital will be lower than the frequency of fits seen in a tertiary-referral neonatal intensive care unit which only admits high-risk, ill infants.

TYPES OF NEONATAL FIT

A variety of different types of neonatal fit are recognized. Infants can present with tonic stiffenings and it may be difficult to distinguish this type of movement from decerebrate posturing or even opisthotonos. Tonic and/or clonic seizures are well known and are unlikely to be missed. Less commonly, convulsions may be of the focal clonic type, involving only one limb and unaccompanied by unconsciousness, and more rarely myoclonic seizures are recognized. The most difficult type of fits to diagnose are the so-called 'subtle seizures' (Volpe, 1981), because they can appear to be simply the features seen in any ill neonate. The only manifestation of subtle seizures may be tonic deviation of the eyes, blinking, lip-smacking or apnoeic spells. Apnoea itself is not infrequently due to a seizure disorder, and it can be extremely difficult to distinguish the cause of the apnoea which commonly occurs in compromised infants. Apnoea occurring in neurologically compromised infants may be the only feature of seizure activity. Abnormal movements related to involvement of the basal ganglia characteristically include 'swimming' movements of the arms or 'cycling' movements of the legs. These types of seizure are not uncommonly seen. The observer's level of suspicion for diagnosing convulsions influences the reported frequency of this condition. The more immature the infant, the less typical will the seizures be and the more difficult will it be to make a confident diagnosis.

CONTINUOUS EEG MONITORING

Recently, continuous electroencephalographic (EEG) monitoring has become available (Bjerre et al., 1983; Eyre et al., 1983) and it is now possible to monitor electroseizure activity for days at a time. Two methods exist: the cerebral function monitor (Bjerre et al., 1983), and the Oxford Instruments' 24-hour EEG tape system (Eyre et al., 1983). The latter is a more reliable instrument in that it is less prone to movement artefact. The Oxford workers have shown that, of 25 infants with electroseizure activity as diagnosed by continuous EEG monitoring, only 13 (54%) showed abnormal movements of any type and only eight (32%) had typical clonic or tonic seizures (Eyre et al., 1983). Relying on clinical criteria for diagnosing seizures will grossly underestimate their frequency.

INCIDENCE

The incidence of neonatal seizures (per 1000 live births) has been variously reported as 1.5 (Eriksson and Zetterstrom, 1979), 3.7 (Gentz et al., 1969), 8.6 (Goldberg, 1983) and 14 (Brown et al., 1972). There is some evidence that the frequency of neonatal convulsions has risen in recent years. Studies from Melbourne, Australia, have shown an increase from two per 1000 in 1971–4 to

8.6 per 1000 in 1978–80 (Goldberg, 1983). The suggested reason for this increase is more referrals of high-risk pregnancies and babies to specialized perinatal units.

AETIOLOGY

The major causes of seizures include birth asphyxia, intracranial haemorrhage, metabolic disturbances, meningo-encephalitis, development abnormalities of the brain, and narcotic withdrawal. The latter is uncommon in most centres in this country but is commonly seen in the United States. However, there seems to be a popular misconception that neonatal convulsions occur commonly in babies who are withdrawing from their maternal opiate state, whereas the reported incidence of neonatal convulsions in babies born to addicted mothers lies between 1 and 3%; extreme jitteriness and irritability on the other hand are frequently seen. In addition, most published reports include a large group in which no cause can be found. In some centres, notably Melbourne, up to one-third of infants have benign seizures on or about the fifth day of life and this has been referred to as 'fifth-day fits'. The cause of these seizures is not clear and it has been suggested that central nervous system zinc deficiency is an important factor (Goldberg and Sheehy, 1982).

There are few reports giving the incidence of causes of neonatal convulsions. Table I shows causes reported in two recent papers. The largest group was either asphyxia or idiopathic convulsions in which no definite cause could be found. I have included 'fifth-day fitters' in this group in view of their uncertain nature. Infection, hypoglycaemia, hypocalcaemia, metabolic disorders and intracranial haemorrhage were rarer causes for neonatal convulsions.

INTRACRANIAL HAEMORRHAGE

In the last few years high-quality ultrasound has become available for scanning the newborn brain (Levene *et al.*, 1985). All full-term infants admitted to the

Table I   Causes of neonatal convulsions (expressed as a percentage of the total) in three different centres

	Stockholm (Eriksson and Zetterstrom, 1979) $N = 77$	Melbourne (Goldberg, 1983) $N = 235$	Leicester (1984) $N = 46$
Unknown cause	28	48	4
Asphyxia	47	31	52
Infection	12	5	7
Hypoglycaemia	7	2	4
Hypocalcaemia	3	6	0
Metabolic disorders	3	3	7
Haemorrhage	0	3	17
Other	0	2	9

Leicester Royal Infirmary with convulsions in the first month of life and who underwent full investigations, including a brain scan, were reviewed. A cause for the convulsion was found in 96% of cases. Asphyxia was the commonest cause (52%), but haemorrhage was found in 17%. These included four cases of intraventricular haemorrhage, one of primary intracerebral haemorrhage, two of thalamic and one of subarachnoid bleeding.

Bleeding into the ventricles can occur from a number of sites: the primary choroid-plexus bleed occurs in full-term asphyxiated babies and the seizures usually start within the first 24 hours. One infant presented with purpura and seizures; his mother had idiopathic thrombocytopenic purpura and he had massive bilateral intracerebral haemorrhage. Primary intracerebral haemorrhage related to the ventricles is not common. In one of the four cases we have seen there was primary intrathalamic haemorrhage in a full-term infant who, having appeared completely normal and been discharged home, presented at between 10 and 14 days with seizures. There were characteristic eye signs – deviation of the eyes downwards and to the side of the thalamic haemorrhage, which can be explained on the basis of the neuroanatomy of the visual pathway. This condition follows a remarkably consistent course that can usually be recognized in the first instance without recourse to imaging techniques. These babies normally make good progress (Trounce et al., 1985).

In addition three other infants with fits were found to have sustained cerebral arterial infarction. If scanning had not been available these 11 cases would probably have been described as idiopathic.

Subdural haemorrhage can also give rise to seizures. Babies who are asphyxiated are at risk of other intracranial problems; we therefore scan all asphyxiated infants and recognize haemorrhage or ischaemic disorders not uncommonly. If subdural haemorrhage is suspected, CT scanning is a better imaging technique than ultrasound to detect these lesions, which may require further treatment. Tentorial tear can also be associated with subdural bleeding and seizures: it used to be thought that this condition carried a high mortality rate, but it is now recognized that tentorial tear with associated haemorrhage is not uncommon following asphyxia and may be diagnosed by ultrasound or on CT scanning.

CONCLUSION

In summary, neonatal seizures are a common condition, with a wide variety of causes, of which asphyxia is the most common. Modern imaging techniques have considerably improved our ability to assign a cause to the seizures, and intracranial haemorrhage is now the second most common condition predisposing to convulsions in the neonatal period. More precise diagnosis will allow a more accurate prediction of outcome.

REFERENCES

BJERRE, I., HELLSTON-WESTAS, L., ROSEN, I., and SVENNINGSEN, N. (1983) Monitoring of cerebral function after severe asphyxia in infancy. *Arch. Dis. Child.*, **58**, 997–1002.

BROWN, J. K., COCKBURN, F., and FORFAR, J. O. (1972) Clinical and chemical correlates in convulsions of the newborn. *Lancet i*, 135–139.

ERIKSSON, M., and ZETTERSTROM, R. (1979) Neonatal convulsions. Incidence and causes in the Stockholm area. *Acta Paediatr. Scand.*, **68**, 807–811.

EYRE, J. A., OOZEER, R. C., and WILKINSON, A. R. (1983) Diagnosis of neonatal seizures by continuous recording and rapid analysis of the electroencephalogram. *Arch. Dis. Child.*, **58**, 785–790.

GENTZ, J., PERRSON, B., and ZETTERSTROM, R. (1969) On the diagnosis of symptomatic neonatal hypoglycaemia. *Acta Paediatr. Scand.*, **58**, 449–452.

GOLDBERG, H. J. (1983) Neonatal convulsions – a 10-year review. *Arch. Dis. Child.*, **58**, 976–978.

GOLDBERG, H. J., and SHEEHY, E. M. (1982) Fifth-day fits: an acute zinc deficiency syndrome? *Arch. Dis. Child.*, **57**, 633–635.

LEVENE, M. I., WILLIAMS, J. L., and FAWER, C.-L. (1985) *Ultrasound Scanning of the Infant Brain*. Spastics International Medical Publications, London.

TROUNCE, J. Q., DODD, K. L., FAWER, C.-L., FIELDER, A. R., PUNT, J., and LEVENE, M. I. (1985) Primary thalamic haemorrhage in the newborn: A new clinical entity. *Lancet i*, 190–192.

VOLPE, J. J. (1981) *Neurology of the Newborn*. W. B. Saunders, Philadelphia.

Paediatric Perspectives on Epilepsy
Edited by E. Ross and E. Reynolds
© 1985 John Wiley & Sons Ltd.

3

The prognosis and management of neonatal seizures

B. G. R. NEVILLE
Guy's Hospital, London

SUMMARY

The prognosis of neonatal seizures ranges from very poor, where the cause is hypoxic-ischaemic damage, to very good in babies with benign fifth-day seizures and seizures caused by a simple metabolic disorder like hypocalcaemia. The extent of intervention, therefore, is partly dependent upon prognosis where the cause is apparent. Important recent advances in the understanding of pharmacokinetics of anticonvulsant drugs in the newborn period suggest that same-day anticonvulsant levels are essential for management. The spectrum of pyridoxine dependency has been widened. The management of epilepsy in the newborn period is an integral part of intensive care, and the value of continuous physiological and EEG monitoring is emerging from a number of studies.

INTRODUCTION

The newborn make up a very important group of patients with epilepsy, calling for particular attention to prognosis, diagnosis, multiplicity of causes, pyridoxine dependency and drug treatment.

PROGNOSIS

It is impossible to consider the management of seizures in the newborn without taking into account what is known about outcome. In neonates the general prognostic principles of childhood epilepsy also apply, the outcome being progressively poorer in those children with evidence of additional cerebral handicaps. However, where seizures are of a simple type and occur as an isolated phenomenon, often time-locked, stimulus-provoked, and with a strong genetic component, the outcome is usually very good indeed. Both extremes are represented in the newborn period, the former occurring in babies with prenatal and hypoxic-ischaemic damage and the latter in those with fifth-day seizures and simple hypocalcaemia.

Global figures in the newborn period need to be read with care because these causes vary in frequency and because in the studies that have been published different criteria are used for age at presentation, gestational age and place of birth.

Goldberg, in a 10-year study from Melbourne, showed an incidence rising from two to 8.6 per 1000 live births and in only 11% of his series was the cause unknown (Goldberg, 1983). Fifth-day seizures were regarded as a known cause and, with hypoxic-ischaemic damage, were the commonest. The steady mortality of about 50% in the hypoxic-ischaemic group indicates the severity of the damage preceding the seizures. Although this implies a hope that effective treatment of seizures may mitigate the outcome, we have no clear evidence that this is happening yet. Within the hypoxic-ischaemic group there is evidence that those with clinical seizures do relatively worse, only 10% in one series having a normal outcome.

In the Edinburgh series, 50% of babies with hypoxic-ischaemic damage had clinical seizures (Brown et al., 1974) and there is evidence (see below) that a further 25% of such babies may be having subclinical seizures. Another useful figure from that study was that only 8% of such babies had epilepsy as their sole manifestation of brain dysfunction.

Dennis, in her study from Oxford, separated prenatal from perinatal causes and affirmed an important clinical sign: that a positively normal neonatal discharge assessment was a predictor of a good outcome (Dennis, 1978).

There seems very little justification for separating the prognosis of early-onset epilepsy in neurologically abnormal babies from that of prenatal and perinatal brain malformation and that of intrapartum asphyxia.

Dennis also gave 20–25% for the late incidence of epilepsy in the non-metabolic group, that is, the expected rate for their degree of handicap, which is usually a combination of mental handicap and spastic quadriplegia.

THE DIAGNOSIS OF NEONATAL SEIZURES

Problems are mostly encountered in babies who are sick and asphyxiated. Brown et al. (1974) and Volpe (1983) have described the sequence of neurological signs that tends to follow such an event, with seizures usually beginning at between 6 and 24 hours. The fragmentary nature of the attacks is well known.

A number of studies have shown that the electroencephalogram (EEG) may show evidence of dysrhythmia as a sole manifestation in significant numbers

(Eyre *et al.*, 1983). Major cardiovascular abnormalities, including ventricular tachycardia occurring with such EEG phenomena and responding to anticonvulsants, have been described. There are sufficient data from animal studies to suggest that it is worth stopping brain dysrhythmias in a baby who is pharmacologically or pathologically paralysed.

The situation occasionally arises in which primitive motor patterns may be mistaken for seizures. For example, babies with the Prader–Willi syndrome may have episodes of eye-rolling and stiffening which can be misleading, particularly if the baby's hypotonia is regarded as secondary to hypoxia. Also, a baby may present with a condition such as Menkes's syndrome in which fits can be confidently predicted. Babies with an intrauterine cause for their epilepsy are very likely also to have intrauterine seizures which may be of much greater significance to the developing brain.

THE MULTIPLICITY OF CAUSES

Table I lists the investigations useful for determining which of the many possible causes is responsible. It is important to recognize that the rare metabolic causes of acute encephalopathies which often include seizures, and which are dependent upon the ingestion of a normal diet (for example, the hyperammonaemic syndromes), tend to present around the age of 24 hours with an unexpected acute illness which is often mistaken for infection. It is important, in addition to treating for infection, that protein and galactose are withdrawn from the diet and that metabolic investigations are performed without delay.

Table I   Investigations of use in neonatal seizures

	Investigations
Blood	Glucose concentration; sugar chromatography; calcium and magnesium levels; electrolytes, osmolality; concentrations of bilirubin, gases, ammonia, amino acids; culture; drug levels; screening for intrauterine infection
Urine	Concentration of amino acids, sugars, organic acids
Ultrasound	
Cerebrospinal fluid	Routine
Intravenous pyridoxine	
Maternal drug status and fetal heart rate	
Computerized tomography of head	
Chromosomes	
(Neurological intensive care)	

Rose and Lombroso (1970) have pointed out that hypocalcaemia and hypermagnesaemia are found in asphyxiated babies in the first two days of life.

The combination of respiratory, infective and metabolic causes of seizures in asphyxiated premature babies is well known. An important advance has been made in recognizing the increased sodium requirements of premature babies (Al-Dahhan *et al.*, 1983) because of the close relationship between hyponatraemia and cerebral oedema.

The management of newborn convulsions is therefore an intensive-care rather than a purely neurological exercise.

PYRIDOXINE-DEPENDENT EPILEPSY

Although this autosomal recessive disorder is very rare it is often worth bearing in mind. The important new points about this disorder are:

(a) It may previously have been missed in a baby who died with seizures.

(b) Neonates with pyridoxine dependency may have intrapartum asphyxia. It is thus wrong to assume that asphyxia *per se* was the cause of the fit, and a trial of pyridoxine is always indicated in these cases.

(c) The neurological findings or EEG may not be immediately restored to normal by pyridoxine, and therefore a remission may only be recognized in retrospect.

(d) A dose of 100 mg intravenously is usually used. One baby that we treated became rapidly flaccid and we discovered that this was a recognized phenomenon (Kroll, 1985). Therefore resuscitation facilities are much more important than an EEG.

(e) In an interesting study from Melbourne, some babies were found to have a brief response to traditional anticonvulsants; it was also found that seizures may start as late as six weeks of age (Bankier *et al.*, 1983).

(f) The outcome is generally poor, with a high incidence of mental handicap; however, in one family known to us in which three children were affected the outcome became progressively better the earlier treatment was started. It is interesting to speculate that the epilepsy rate in this handicapped group of survivors may be lower than expected.

THE DRUG MANAGEMENT OF
EPILEPSY IN THE NEWBORN

The unusual pharmacokinetics and problems of achieving effective blood levels rapidly have led to some misapprehensions about the value of individual drugs. The reason so few good trials have been carried out may be partly because of the problem of controlling for the many variables.

There is a very good review of these problems in *Recent Advances in Epilepsy* (Dodson, 1983). Although many drugs are used, only those in most common use will be discussed here.

Phenobarbitone in premature babies may have a half-life of up to 200 hours, which makes any routine scheme of administration meaningless. Maternal ingestion of an *anticonvulsant* acts as a hepatic enzyme inducer in the newborn.

Phenytoin is very effective and in one study nearly 90% of seizures in neonates were controlled. Its early half-life is long but rapidly falls by the end of the first week.

Diazepam is effective but is rapidly lost in fat. It also tends to depress ventilation if repeated doses are given, particularly if other drugs have been used or if cerebral oedema is present. Therefore it is best used as an initial measure.

There does not seem to be much information about the use of *carbamazepine* in neonates. Because of the wide variation in drug handling in sick neonates, same-day blood-level measurements are necessary in all but the simplest situations and intensive-care facilities should also be available.

Lastly, *thiopentone* is totally effective but masks all the physical signs.

The doses quoted in Table II (Dodson, 1983) may seem rather high but it seems likely that they are close to the loading doses required for phenobarbitone and phenytoin.

Table II   Intravenous (i.v.) or intramuscular (i.m.) dosages of drugs in common use for the treatment of seizures in the newborn (Dodson, 1983)

Drug	Initial dose	Initial daily maintenance
Calcium gluconate (10%)	2 ml/kg i.v.	1 mmol/kg/day
Diazepam	0.5 mg/kg i.v.	Not repeated
Glucose (25%)	2–4 ml/kg i.v.	0.5 mg/kg/hour
Magnesium sulphate (50%)	0.2 ml/kg i.m.	0.2 ml/kg
Phenobarbitone	20 mg/kg i.v.	3.5 mg/kg
Phenytoin	20 mg/kg i.v.	8 mg/kg

The final question to be considered is the major problem of the content and use of neurological intensive care. It is possible to have available: continuous EEG, intracranial pressure monitoring with blood pressure and continuous cerebral perfusion pressure, middle cerebral bloodflow, continuous oxygen and CO_2, and evoked responses. This highly labour-intensive monitoring should in my view be used as a research technique to decide on the best non-invasive techniques for routine use.

Several problems remain unanswered in the hypoxic-ischaemic group of babies:

(a) Does dysrhythmia damage the brain?
(b) Does maintaining cerebral perfusion help outcome?
(c) What is the influence of sodium balance on outcome?
(d) Do drugs minimize damage? and
(e) Are our efforts too late?

In my opinion, for routine management careful standard physiological monitoring plus continuous EEG may be the best compromise at present.

Many problems therefore remain in our attitude to seizures in the poor-outcome group. The high morbidity and mortality in babies with hypoxic-ischaemic damage continues in the face of increasingly vigorous treatment of seizures; if it conceals a consequence of our intervention, it certainly does so very effectively.

REFERENCES

AL-DAHHAN, J., HAYCOCK, G. B., CHANTLER, C., and STIMMLER, L. (1983) Sodium homeostasis in term and preterm neonates. 1. Renal aspects. Arch. Dis. Child., 58, 335–342.

BANKIER, A., TURNER, M., and HOPKINS, I. J. (1983) Pyridoxine-dependent seizures – a wider clinical spectrum. Arch. Dis. Child., 58, 415–418.

BROWN, J. K., PURVIS, R. J., FORFAR, J. O., and COCKBURN, F. (1974) Neurologic aspects of perinatal asphyxia. Dev. Med. Child Neurol., 16, 567–580.

DENNIS, J. (1978) Neonatal convulsions: aetiology, late neonatal status and long-term outcome. Dev. Med. Child Neurol., 20, 143–158.

DODSON, E. (1983) Antiepileptic drug use in newborn and infants. In: Recent Advances in Epilepsy, pp. 231–248 (Eds T. A. Pedley and B. S. Meldrum). Churchill Livingstone, Edinburgh.

EYRE, J. A. OOZEER, R. C., and WILKINSON, A. R. (1983) Diagnosis of neonatal seizures by continuous recording and rapid analysis of the electroencephalogram. Arch. Dis. Child., 58, 785–790.

GOLDBERG, H. J. (1983) Neonatal convulsions – a 10-year review. Arch. Dis. Child., 58, 976–978.

GOLDBERG, R. N., GOLDMAN, S. L., RAMSAY, R. E., and FELLER, R. (1982) Detection of seizure activity in the paralysed neonate using continuous monitoring. Pediatrics, 69, 583–586.

KROLL, J. S. (1985) The trial of pyridoxine in neonatal seizures: an unexpected danger. Dev. Med. Child Neurol., 27, in press.

ROSE, A. L., and LOMBROSO, C. T. (1970) Neonatal seizure states. A study of clinical, pathological and electroencephalographic features in 137 full-term babies with a long-term follow-up. Pediatrics, 45, 404–425.

VOLPE, J. J. (1983) Perinatal hypoxic-ischaemic brain injury. Pediatr. Clin. North Am., 23, 383–397.

Discussion

Dr S. H. Green (Birmingham): Professor O'Donohoe, you have talked very clearly about the aetiology of epilepsy. What about the aetiology of individual seizures? Do you believe that each individual seizure must be in response to an environmental influence, or are some seizures in predisposed individuals truly random events? And should we be looking more carefully for the causes of each individual seizure?

O'Donohoe: It would be an impossible task to look at each individual seizure. But certainly where a child has stayed seizure free for months or even years and then had a seizure, the cause should be sought in environmental or biological factors operating at the time. This is particularly true of adolescents who have omitted their drugs, or stayed up all night, or something of that order. One should look critically at the seizure that is out of context.

Dr M. R. Trimble (London): In your paper you referred to lesions, but are there lesions in many of these cases? If not, what are the functional changes that provoke a seizure? And when you say lesion, what are you actually referring to? In many cases of epilepsy we see no lesion in pathological specimens.

O'Donohoe: I use the term lesional the way Henri Gastaut does – to indicate some sort of structural change, either inherited or acquired. Consider, for example, benign partial rolandic epilepsy, which deserves great study. Why do so many children with it sometimes have very frequent EEG discharges and maybe only one or two seizures? Something must trigger off the seizures, and some people have suggested that there may be an underlying lesion as well, a structural lesion. But maybe it is bad to use a definite term for something so uncertain.

Dr. R. O. Robinson (London): We have to recognize that all neurones have intrinsic burst capabilities which look remarkably like excitatory post-synaptic potentials. Perhaps we should think of the brain as being in a constant state of barely suppressed activity. Seizures could be triggered by failure to suppress this tonic intrinsic burst capability, i.e. by sudden disinhibition. The parts of the brain which are most easily fired into epileptogenic activity—the hippocampus and three or four areas of the cortex—are those most richly supplied with GABA-ergic endings. This is in line with our understanding of how anticonvulsants work, by modifying the GABA-ergic receptors. So perhaps we should begin to think about 'lesions' affecting these mechanisms.

Dr S. Rose (Inverness): It is said that an infant with fits may not have an abnormal EEG, and that an abnormal tracing suggestive of epilepsy may not be associated with fits. Yet in neonates, if I understand correctly, we are advised to try and control such EEG abnormalities by treatment, and animal work is said to support this view. But are we really expected to monitor all neonates and treat those with EEG signs? Or should we still trust our clinical judgement and only treat fits in infants who jerk?

Dr E. M. Ross (London): You've got the very nub of the argument. On one hand, we're saying treat all fits vigorously because of the kindling theory; on the other, we say don't treat certain types of fit, such as nocturnal ones.

Levene: This is a very important question. Basically we're talking about different things. One is how to treat a fitting baby in hospital; at the moment, all we can do is to treat symptomatic seizures. The most important thing, however, is the baby's condition between seizures. The more neurologically abnormal he is between seizures, the more important it is to investigate and to orientate care around the baby's cerebral function. If the baby is having occasional seizures and appears to be entirely normal between them, as the fifth-day fitters are, then it's probably not essential to control fits in the way that you would try to in a baby who was neurologically abnormal. Several centres are studying continuous EEG monitoring to try and answer these questions. If babies are having epileptic discharges without showing seizure activity, does this matter? Do such discharges damage the brain? If so, how can they best be controlled? The answer to the first question is that we do not know, but there is animal evidence that continuous abnormal discharges are probably harmful. The answer to the second question is even more difficult because we cannot control the abnormal discharges in many of these neurologically abnormal babies with the anticonvulsant drugs currently in use. We are therefore beginning to explore the effect of some newer anticonvulsants. This is very much a research area at the moment. When controlled studies are completed, they may show the best way of treating these seizures and whether treatment makes any difference to the long-term prognosis.

Professor O. Eeg-Olofsson (Linköping): I was very impressed by Professor O'Donohoe's dynamic approach to the aetiology of epilepsy. Among the multifactorial influences at work, there might be an immune deficiency mechanism in the benign epilepsy of children with temporo-central spikes and shock waves. I have found a low frequency of HLA A_1B_8 in this group and in their parents. This is the most common HLA type in our general population, and the low frequency in these epileptic children suggests that it may confer some biological advantage, perhaps as a protector mechanism against infectious disease. In other words, the children prone to this type of epilepsy may be subject to some kind of immune deficiency. Interestingly, I also found a decreased frequency of A_1B_8 among patients with focal epilepsy studied in Montreal. However, children with absence epilepsy have a normal frequency of that HLA type. Possibly there is a difference in this respect between the generalized and the focal types of epileptic disorder.

Finally, a question to Dr Levene. Behind your high figure of 54% asphyxia in the Leicester study, there must be many brain malformations; do you think that magnetic resonance imaging will still further reduce the 6% of unknown cause?

Levene: Imaging is a very exciting technique, but there are methodological problems. The scanning is just too slow for critically ill babies to be put into the machine. With time, it may help more. NMR spectroscopy may have more to offer at present, by making it possible to study the biochemical function of the brain; looking at the ratio of ATP to breakdown products can show whether suppressing seizures, either electrically or clinically by means of drugs, actually improves the physiological functioning of the brain. Some new continuously-applied *in vitro* biochemical tests may also help. As far as structural abnormalities are concerned, imaging techniques are certainly getting better.

Dr B. D. Bower (Oxford): Brian Neville referred to Jenny Dennis's follow-up on neonatal convulsions. This cohort is now a decade and a half old and she is still following them up. One of the categories she introduced was 'fetus with a problem', which I have found quite useful. Although it was and is a rather mixed aetiological bag of factors compromising fetal health, it includes almost one-third of the newborns who had seizures. Some are small-for-dates, some have cerebral malformations, others have suggestive pregnancy history. I would like to ask Dr Levene whether he finds an undue proportion of small-for-dates babies in his group of neonatal convulsions who had thalamic haemorrhage after discharge?

Secondly, was there any question of non-accidental abuse in the babies? Could compression of the thorax have raised venous pressure and so put pressure on the thalamus?

Levene: The answer to your first question is that 25% of our babies who suffered from what we call post-asphyxic encephalopathy were growth retarded. In other babies with neonatal seizures, the origin is certainly prenatal, too. The answer to your second question is that we looked very carefully for evidence of non-accidental injury and could find no suspicion of it at all. We looked for a number of different causes, including bleeding disorders, AV malformations and tumours; bleeding from a tumour in the first year of life is probably more common than from an AV malformation. We could find no primary cause in any of these babies. They were all entirely healthy and had been home for at least a week when they presented very acutely with vomiting, bulging fontanelles, hydrocephalus, deviant eye signs and seizures. They follow a remarkably similar clinical and imaging pattern, which has not been described before, but we could find no obvious cause.

Part II: Fits in the remainder of the first year

Paediatric Perspectives on Epilepsy
Edited by E. Ross and E. Reynolds
© 1985 John Wiley & Sons Ltd.

4

The malignant epilepsies of childhood: West's syndrome and the Lennox–Gastaut syndrome

J. K. BROWN and J. LIVINGSTON
Royal Hospital for Sick Children, Edinburgh

SUMMARY

Many seizure disorders in childhood tend to be self-limiting, with a generally good prognosis. These relatively benign epilepsies include petit mal 'absences', febrile convulsions, neonatal seizures due to reversible metabolic disturbances (e.g. hypocalcaemia), and so-called benign rolandic seizures. Brain development is usually unaffected, and at least 80% of such children eventually lead normal lives.

In the so-called malignant epilepsies of childhood – West's syndrome and the Lennox–Gastaut syndrome – at least 80% of sufferers have a continuing handicap throughout childhood and into adult life. West's syndrome consists of infantile (or 'salaam') spasms usually starting in the first year of life, and often associated with hypsarrhythmia in the EEG and mental retardation. Between 20 and 30% of affected children later develop the Lennox–Gastaut syndrome. Its onset typically consists of minor motor seizures ('stare, jerk and fall') in a child aged between two and six years. Slow spike and wave activity in the EEG, associated with mental handicap (in 80–90%) and failure to respond to conventional anticonvulsants are other characteristic features. The Lennox–Gastaut syndrome accounts for over 70% of cases of intractable childhood epilepsy.

WEST'S SYNDROME

The term West's syndrome has become generally accepted to describe a constellation of clinical features consisting of an infantile spasm type of seizure associated with a hypsarrhythmic EEG, a high incidence of mental retardation, and responsiveness to corticosteroid drugs (Table I). Dr West first described

Table I   Main features of West's syndrome

Infantile spasm type of seizure
Mean age 5 months
Hypsarrhythmic EEG
Response to corticosteroids
High incidence of mental handicap
Low genetic proclivity
Periods of minor status with autism and polymyoclonia

the spasms and poor prognosis in his own child in 1841 in a letter to the *Lancet*. Diagnostic difficulty arises in that only some 66% of children with infantile spasms have a hypsarrhythmic EEG. They may not have mental retardation and in certain subgroups the response to ACTH is poor. The infantile spasm type of seizure is occasionally seen in normal infants with a normal EEG and no mental retardation (Gastaut *et al.*, 1964; Jeavons and Bower, 1964; Lacy and Penry, 1976).

In 90% of cases of West's syndrome the spasms start in the first year of life, and only very rarely commence after two years. Most commence in the three- to nine-month age period, with a peak between four and six months. Many authors have found a male preponderance, but this is not consistent enough to be of diagnostic or aetiological importance. The incidence is low, only one in 3000, compared with 100 in 3000 for pyrexial convulsions. A positive family history is unusual in the sense of the inherited propensity to 3 Hz synchrony and generalization, but may be obtained in cases with genetic disease, e.g. tuberous sclerosis. Infantile spasms are age specific and dependent upon the stage of brain maturation. The high incidence of associated long-term handicap and mental retardation reflects the severity of the brain damage necessary to produce fits at this age. The syndrome can be regarded as a brainstem release phenomenon resulting from diffuse or multifocal neocortical damage.

Clinical features

The infantile spasm, salaam attacks or lightning spasm develops in a previously normal infant (Zellweger, 1948) in about 40% of cases, whilst in 60% it is symptomatic, the infant having previously shown abnormal development. This division has become less crisp since modern imaging techniques have made it possible to demonstrate pre-existing genetic pathology in many cases. The infant may have presented with a seizure disorder at birth or may have developed focal, i.e. partial, seizures with simple symptomatology around six weeks of age, associated with subsequent change to a classical infantile spasm.

In a typical spasm there is involvement of axial and limb musculature. The classical lightning spasm is a sudden jerk lasting less than two seconds;

sometimes there is a tonic spasm when the movement appears to 'hang up' for between two and 10 seconds. The spasm is followed by a period of no movement, the infant may cry with the spasm, appear to be in discomfort or, less commonly, smile. Kellaway *et al.* (1983) pointed out that there are three types of spasm: *flexor*, in 34% of cases; *extensor*, in 23%, and *mixed*, in 42%. In the classical flexor spasm there may simply be head flexion, i.e. a head nod difficult to recognize unless one is aware of its restricted nature. More typically, the head flexes, the knees pull up, the arms suddenly flex, the abdominal muscles contract and the baby goes into complete flexion of neck, trunk, arms and legs, jack-knifing at the waist. These episodes are very similar to startle responses.

The extensor spasm is in effect a Moro reflex, in which the arms suddenly abduct and extend, the neck and trunk extend, and the legs extend; difficulty may be encountered in differentiating this type of spasm from dystonic attacks in the brain-damaged child. The mixed picture consists, for example, of the arms and head flexing and the legs extending. One could regard these seizures as a release of primitive reflexes. The seizures are more likely to occur when the infant is awakening or going to sleep and tend to come in bursts, but are not repeated in rapid succession; there is usually 30 seconds to one minute between spasms. The infant may have anything from five to 100 over the course of a day. In a bout, the intervals gradually get longer and the spasms less forceful, before they die away. In most infants, handling, noise, light and feeding do not precipitate the seizure, but there are a minority in whom the spasm appears as a reflex seizure, e.g. when trying to elicit a plantar response.

The onset of the spasms may be associated with an apparent loss of abilities, the child appearing vacant and less responsive. Polymyoclonic movements of the fingers (repeated small flexor and extensor) also occur. These features accompanying classical flexor spasms leave no doubt about the diagnosis. But sudden abdominal stiffening or jack-knifing, pulling up the knees, or head nods may suggest simple colic or an abdominal catastrophe, such as intussusception.

Aetiology

Just under half of all cases of West's syndrome are cryptogenic, i.e. there does not appear to be any obvious cause. The infant will have developed absolutely normally until the time when the seizures appear. In this group the response to steroids is usually excellent and the prognosis for future mental handicap is much better than in the symptomatic group. The main pathology in symptomatic infantile spasms appears to consist of extensive bilateral and multifocal lesions in the cerebral hemispheres (Rukonen and Donner, 1979).

This can be due to infection, which may be prenatal (cytomegalovirus or toxoplasmosis) or postnatal (virus encephalitis). The possibility of postnatal infection with cytomegalovirus should also be borne in mind. Brain damage from perinatal events, especially asphyxia, is a common cause of infantile spasms, following a latent period of apparent recovery from the perinatal problems. Low birth weight has been associated with infantile spasms (Crichton, 1968). Like infection and asphyxia, congenital malformations can cause multiple or diffuse cortical lesions, and these form the third main aetiological group. West's syndrome can also occur in infants with known metabolic diseases such as phenylketonuria, Krabbe's leucodystrophy, Leigh's encephalopathy, or non-ketotic hyperglycinaemia. Any cerebral pathology may have preceded the onset, including non-accidental injury, subdural haematoma, head injury, and tumours of the meninges. At present, there is no clear evidence about the possible aetiological role of pertussis immunization.

Investigation

Computerized tomography (CT) is of value in the diagnosis of anatomical abnormalities or calcification, e.g. agenesis of the corpus callosum (Gastaut *et al.*, 1978) and tuberous sclerosis (Kuhlendahl *et al.*, 1977). About a quarter of all children with West's syndrome have a normal CT scan. The most common finding is cerebral atrophy, but its significance is open to question if steroid therapy has been started, as this can produce similar appearances due to reduction in brain water.

The classical EEG finding is hypsarrhythmia (Gibbs *et al.*, 1954), present in two-thirds of cases. This consists of randomized slow waves with no synchrony, which are of high voltage, with completely random epileptic spike activity, which is not propagated, from all parts of the cortex. During actual spasm, the EEG flattens and does not show a sudden increase in spikes. Although the clinical infantile spasm and hypsarrhythmia are considered integral parts of West's syndrome, they are not interdependent (Watanabe *et al.*, 1973). As the child gets older, hypsarrhythmia tends to synchronize more and may gradually merge into the gross spike-wave phenomena of the Lennox–Gastaut syndrome. Several other EEG patterns may be seen in West's syndrome, including focal spikes, normal tracings, or a burst suppression pattern similar to that normally seen in non-eye-movement sleep in a full-term baby. When hypsarrhythmia is associated with West's syndrome, the child may turn out to be mentally normal. Or a child with infantile spasms but no hypsarrhythmia may have severe brain damage with subsequent mental and physical handicap. Treatment may reduce spasms or hypsarrhythmia, independently of each other.

Treatment

Conventional anticonvulsant drugs are ineffective against infantile spasms. The two most effective methods of treatment are steroids or enhancement of GABA inhibition (Sorel and Dusaucy-Bauloye, 1958; Klein and Livingston, 1950; Pavone *et al.*, 1981). It is difficult to know how ACTH or adrenal steroids exert their effect in infantile spasms and hypsarrhythmia. Kellaway *et al.* (1983) find that steroids have an all or none effect, there being no partial control of infantile spasms or hypsarrhythmia. Most centres give 20–40 units of ACTH in gel form, daily for a month, and then substitute prednisolone in reducing dosage over a further two months. Others give ACTH for six months or oral prednisolone or dexamethasone from the start. ACTH is dramatic in stopping the fits in 70% of cases and returns the EEG to normal in about 40%. About 37% of the children get steroid side effects, and 5% mortality has been attributed to them. Unfortunately, cessation of the seizures and normalization of the EEG does not seem to have any influence on the long-term prognosis, particularly of *symptomatic* infantile spasms. And the initial improvement in seizures and hypsarrhythmia may not hold. Most paediatricians start benzodiazepine therapy during the course of steroids, rather than risk a later return of seizures. Benzodiazepine therapy is discussed in more detail in the section on Lennox–Gastaut syndrome (page 36).

Prognosis

The outlook for children with West's syndrome is very poor. At least 80% become mentally handicapped, with a smaller percentage of perhaps 50% in the cryptogenic group. About 10% die, and 25% also have some form of cerebral palsy. The prognosis depends on whether development is normal at the onset, and upon the aetiology, in that gross cortical dysplasia or tuberous sclerosis, for example, can be expected to show the prognosis of the disease. Many of the children, apart from being mentally retarded, also show autistic features (Jeavons *et al.*, 1970; Matsumoto *et al.*, 1981; Kurokawa *et al.*, 1980). At least half will continue with another form of seizure disorder. The infantile spasm type of seizure usually disappears by three years of age, and the EEG changes as the brain matures, from hypsarrhythmia to a more generalized spike and wave pattern. In 25–30% of children this merges with the Lennox–Gastaut syndrome, so that an intractable seizure disorder persists into later childhood. In a large Japanese series of infantile spasms, completely normal mental and physical development was achieved in less than 10% (Matsumoto *et al.*, 1981).

The poor prognostic factors were identified as: relapse after ACTH therapy, epileptic seizures concomitant with infantile spasms, and a different type of seizure disorder preceding the onset of spasms. In cryptogenic cases, there was a significant correlation between delay in treatment and a poor long-term prognosis for mental development. However, Jeavons and Bower (1961) studied 30 infants, none of whom were treated with corticotrophin or steroids, and they found that 50% were free of seizures by three years and one-third had normal EEGs; there was little difference between the symptomatic and cryptogenic group in terms of disappearance of spasms and EEG improvement.

THE LENNOX-GASTAUT SYNDROME

One of the best recognized abnormalities in electroencephalography is the typical 3 Hz spike and wave activity of classical petit mal. In 1939, Gibbs et al. described slower rhythmical spike and wave activity, usually at 2–2.5 Hz, associated with other types of seizure and often with mental retardation (Gibbs and Gibbs, 1962), which became known as 'petit mal variant'. Lennox (1945) subsequently described this association of complex absences associated with other forms of motor seizure, mental retardation and the slower spike or polyspike and wave. After publication of a paper by Gastaut et al. in 1966, which further expanded the syndrome to include the child with epileptic encephalopathy with slow spikes and waves, this became known as the Lennox–Gastaut syndrome. Classically, a child between one and six years of age develops minor motor seizures consisting of absence, myoclonic jerks and akinetic falls, together with a slow spike and wave EEG in the region of 1.5–2.5 Hz, a low genetic propensity, marked drug resistance, and mental handicap in over 85% (Table II).

Table II   Main features of Lennox–Gastaut
syndrome

Minor motor seizures – stare, jerk and fall
EEG shows slow spike and wave activity 1.5–2.5 Hz
Resistant to conventional anticonvulsants
Most mentally handicapped (80–90%)
Episodes of minor 'status' or encephalopathy
Age 2–6 years

This is one of the most malignant forms of epilepsy in childhood, constituting more than 70% of intractable cases. Though probably heterogeneous, it is clinically a very useful group. There is a close link between infantile spasms and the Lennox–Gastaut syndrome, in that one may lead to the other, and both tend to be age-dependent seizure patterns which are not specific in aetiology but characteristic of the stage of development of the nervous system (Aicardi and Chevrie, 1971; Chevrie and Aicardi, 1972; Schneider et al., 1970; Livingston et al., 1958). The Lennox–Gastaut syndrome can persist into adult life, and some severely brain-damaged children may never reach a stage of brain development capable of inhibiting the pattern. This type of seizure disorder is therefore very common in long-stay residents of mental deficiency hospitals.

Aetiology

About 20–30% of children with infantile spasms progress to the Lennox–Gastaut syndrome. In other cases it may be associated with acquired lesions such as head injury, measles encephalitis, anoxia (e.g. from severe prolonged pyrexial convulsions) or lead poisoning (Fejerman *et al.*, 1973), or with degenerative brain disease such as Batten's disease and subacute sclerosing panencephalitis. Some cases appear to be due to a form of subacute encephalopathy. Subacute encephalitis with measles or rubella virus needs to be excluded. It is now recognized that children with intrauterine infections such as rubella, toxoplasmosis and cytomegalovirus may have a progressive encephalopathy, with reactivation of the virus later in childhood. When all of these conditions have been excluded, one is left with a cryptogenic group in previously normal children, about four years old, some of whom remain mentally normal and in whom no cause can be found.

Clinical features

The classical minor motor seizures are best described as 'stare, jerk and fall' epilepsy. The absences or staring attacks may resemble those in petit mal. The jerks are due to sudden myoclonus, which may occur suddenly in an arm or leg (the child may, for example, be sitting at a table and suddenly kick another child, or be thrown off his feet and think he has been pushed). The fall may be due to sudden loss of all postural muscle tone and a true akinetic seizure; at other times it is due to sudden myoclonus or a tonic seizure throwing the child into extension and off balance. Sometimes a minor motor seizure consists of short tonic fits, more likely during sleep. The usual age of seizure onset is between one and six years, in a previously normal child or one handicapped from early infancy.

Between 80% and 90% of affected children are mentally handicapped. This often appears more severe in the toddler and early school years, and may improve somewhat later. Ability appears to be limited by repeated seizures and lack of concentration as well as mental handicap. Major complications are progressive dementia and frequent episodes of minor status epilepticus in some cases (Brett, 1966; Bower, 1972). In these episodes the child appears to switch off from the outside world, and may show more severe autistic features, or become very aggressive. The child may deteriorate in speech, begin to drool and become very wobbly and ataxic. Minor twitchings of the face and hands are reminiscent of the autistic episodes accompanied by polymyoclonia in West's syndrome. Episodes of pseudodementia, ataxia and minor status may last for weeks or months, with dramatic deterioration in behaviour, emotional responsiveness and progress at school.

Children with the Lennox–Gastaut syndrome may have at least 20 minor motor seizures in a 24-hour period, with a range of five to 200 (Papini *et al.*, 1984). Injury from sudden falls is common. Aicardi and Chevrie (1982) have described a more benign variant with a good prognosis, in which the EEG shows a tendency to electrical status during sleep, but this is to some extent a retrospective diagnosis. Doose *et al.* (1970) also described what they call centrencephalic, myoclonic, astatic petit mal when stare, jerk and fall seizures come on in the first five years of life, with progressive dementia. These cases have a very high genetic incidence, and appear to represent a specific disease entity.

Electroencephalography

The classical EEG finding is a spike and wave, synchronous throughout several leads but often not extending equally over both hemispheres, at a frequency between 1.5 and 2.5 Hz. There may be polyspikes rather than a single spike with the wave, best seen in the frontal region and not becoming generalized with every burst. There are often focal or multifocal spikes. The configuration and distribution of successive bursts is not the same, suggesting that there may be generalization from multiple spikes. This would be in keeping with what one would expect if, as brain maturation proceeded from a pattern of hypsarrhythmia, the multiple spike and wave became more organized, more synchronous, and tended to spread after about three years of age. There is no relationship between the EEG and the clinical fit, which need not necessarily occur at the time of the slow spike and wave burst. During tonic fits, the EEG will flatten or a 10 Hz recruiting rhythm may appear. Hypsarrhythmia may persist when the infantile spasms are replaced by stare, jerk and fall seizures. Photic stimulation or hyperventilation will not activate the tendency to generalized spike and wave, seen in the typical 3 Hz discharges of true petit mal. As the slow spike and wave discharge can be associated with other types of seizure (e.g. psychomotor or major tonic-clonic), the diagnosis of Lennox–Gastaut syndrome does not depend upon the EEG findings but on the constellation of abnormalities that make up the whole syndrome.

Treatment

Treatment is very similar to that of West's syndrome, the mainstay being benzodiazepine drugs, steroids or a ketogenic diet, with sodium valproate in a small number of cases. Conventional anticonvulsants such as phenytoin, carbamazepine, phenobarbitone or primidone do not influence the stare, jerk and fall seizures, although a background of major anticonvulsants such as carbamazepine or phenytoin is often maintained to lessen the risk of major tonic-clonic seizures or status epilepticus. In some children, the benzodiazepine drugs used to treat the minor motor seizure may precipitate tonic-clonic seizures or even psychomotor 'status', so carbamazepine is preferred for background maintenance therapy. By eight or nine years of age, the seizure pattern often changes to a mixture of complex partial seizures, generalized major tonic-clonic seizures, and absences; at this stage drugs such as sodium valproate or carbamazepine may be more effective.

Since the seizures are so resistant to conventional anticonvulsant therapy, one must constantly be on the alert against polypharmacy and overdose. It is not unusual to see children on three, four or five anticonvulsants, and there is good evidence that making the child drowsy will greatly increase the number of fits. Papini *et al.* (1984) showed that only 8% of seizures occurred in active wakefulness, compared with 84% when the child was inactively awake or drowsy. If a drug does not reduce the seizures, then it should be discontinued. Drugs such as amphetamine will occasionally improve seizure control. Many other therapies have been tried but none is of proven efficacy (Matsuishi *et al.*, 1983). The insertion of cerebellar pacemakers has a certain theoretical attractiveness, as it is non-destructive and reversible, but results are still inconclusive.

Before starting therapy, we obtain a baseline for the severity of seizures, and test for benzodiazepine sensitivity, which can make dosage very difficult to control. Another problem is habituation, with relapse after several weeks of good control. The benzodiazepines are thought to act by enhancing the sensitivity of the GABA-ergic receptors to endogenous GABA, which is the most potent neurotransmitter inhibitor known.

When steroids are required to control multiple seizures, a short sharp course, similar to that given in infantile spasms, may be effective in 50% of cases (Yamatogi *et al.*, 1979). The EEG, as well as the clinical seizures, will improve with steroid therapy.

For 60 years ketogenic diet has been suggested as a possible measure for managing very severe seizure disorders in young children (Keith, 1963), the idea being to produce ketoacidosis by increasing the amount of fat in the diet and decreasing the amount of carbohydrate. The urine must be checked twice daily, in the morning and evening, to ensure that the child is ketotic, and a multi-vitamin preparation should be given. In certain children the ketogenic diet will have a dramatic effect in reducing the number of seizures, allowing reduction or even cessation of other medication.

In addition to a protective helmet for the child, the family will need a lot of support and help, especially if the medication is not always effective. Side effects may occur and there is always the worry of mental deterioration. Schooling causes difficulties, as intelligence varies quite considerably from week to week, and both teachers and parents need to understand that learning ability varies too, calling for special efforts in the good phases. Behavioural abnormalities, such as overactivity, aggression and a poor emotional response to the parents, can cause more concern than the occurrence of minor motor seizures. In no other area of epileptology does the physician become so aware of his woeful lack of understanding of the mechanisms of the epilepsies and the shortcomings of medication.

REFERENCES

AICARDI, J., and CHEVRIE, J. J. (1971) Myoclonic epilepsies of childhood. *Neuropaediatrie*, **3**, 177–190.
AICARDI, J., and CHEVRIE, J. J. (1982) Atypical benign partial epilepsy of childhood. *Dev. Med. Child Neurol.*, **24**, 281–292.
BOWER, B. D. (1972) Minor epileptic status. *Dev. Med. Child Neurol.*, **14**, 80–81.
BRETT, E. M. (1966) Minor epileptic status. *J. Neurol. Sci.*, **3**, 52–75.
CHEVRIE, J. J., and AICARDI, J. (1972) Childhood epileptic encephalopathy with slow spike wave: A statistical study of 80 cases. *Epilepsia*, **13**, 259–271.
CRICHTON, J. U. (1968) Infantile spasms in children of low birthweight. *Dev. Med. Child Neurol.*, **10**, 36–41.
DOOSE, H., GERKEN, H., LEONHARDT, R., VOLZKE, E., and VOLZ, C. (1970) Centrencephalic myoclonic-astatic petit mal. *Neuropaediatrie*, **2**, 59–78.
FEJERMAN, N., GIMENEZ, E. R., VALLEJO, N. E., and MEDINA, C. S. (1973) Lennox's syndrome and lead intoxication. *Pediatrics*, **52**, 227–234.
GASTAUT, H., ROGER, J., SOULAYROL, R., and PINSARD, N. (1964) *L'Encephalopathie Myoclonique Infantile avec Hypsarhythmie*. Masson, Paris.
GASTAUT, H., ROGER, J., SOULAYROL, R., TASSINARI, C. A., REGIS, H., and DRAVET, C. (1966) Childhood epileptic encephalopathy with diffuse slow spike waves or Lennox syndrome. *Epilepsia*, **7**, 139–179.
GASTAUT, H., GASTAUT, J. L., REGIS, H., BERNARD, R., PINSARD, N., SAINT-JEAN, M., ROGER, J., and DRAVET, C. (1978) Computerised tomography in the study of West's syndrome. *Dev. Med. Child Neurol.*, **20**, 21–27.
GIBBS, E. L., FLEMING, M. M., and GIBBS, F. A. (1954) Diagnosis and prognosis of hypsarrhythmia and infantile spasms. *Pediatrics*, **13**, 66–72.
GIBBS, F. A., and GIBBS, E. L. (1962) *Atlas of Electroencephalography 1962*, **2** (2nd Edn). Addison-Wesley, Reading, Massachusetts.
JEAVONS, P. M., and BOWER, B. D. (1961) The natural history of infantile spasms. *Arch. Dis. Child.*, **36**, 17–22.
JEAVONS, P. M., and BOWER, B. D. (1964) Infantile spasms. A review of the literature and a study of 112 cases. *Clinics in Developmental Medicine*, **No. 15**. Spastics Society with Heinemann Medical, London.
JEAVONS, P. M., HARPER, J. R., and BOWER, B. D. (1970) Long-term prognosis in infantile spasms: a follow-up report on 112 cases. *Dev. Med. Child Neurol.*, **12**, 413–421.
KEITH, H. M. (1963) *Convulsive Disorders in Children with Reference to Treatment with Ketogenic Diet*. Little, Brown, Boston.
KELLAWAY, P., FROST, J. D., and HRACHOVY, R. A. (1983) Infantile spasms. In: *Antiepileptic Drug Therapy in Pediatrics*, pp. 115–136 (Eds P. L. Morselli, C. E. Pippenger and J. K. Penry). Raven Press, New York.
KLEIN, R., and LIVINGSTON, S. (1950) The effect of adreno-corticotrophic hormone in epilepsy. *J. Pediatr.*, **37**, 733–742.
KUHLENDAHL, H. D., GROB-SELBECK, G., DOOSE, H., KLINGE, H., and JENSEN, H. P. (1977) Cranial computer tomography in children with tuberose sclerosis. *Neuropaediatrie*, **8**, 325–332.
KUROKAWA, T., GOYA, N., FUKUYAMA, Y., SUZUKI, M., SEKI, T., and OHTAHARA, S. (1980) West syndrome and Lennox–Gastaut syndrome: A survey of natural history. *Pediatrics*, **65**, 81–88.
LACY, J. R., and PENRY, J. K. (Eds) (1976) *Infantile Spasms*. Raven Press, New York.
LENNOX, W. G. (1945) *Epilepsy and Related Disorders*, **1**. Little, Brown, Boston.

LIVINGSTON, S., EISNER, V., and PAULI, L. (1958) Minor motor epilepsy. Diagnosis, treatment and prognosis. *Pediatrics*, **21**, 916-928.

MATSUISHI, T., YANO, E., INAN AGA, K., TERASAWA, K., ISHIHARA, O., SHIOTSUKI, Y., KATAFUCHI, Y., AOKI, N., and YAMASHITA, F. (1983) A pilot study on the anticonvulsive effects of a thyrotropin-releasing hormone analog in intractable epilepsy. *Brain Dev.*, **5**, 421-428.

MATSUMOTO, A., WATANABE, K., NEGORO, T., SUGUIRA, M., IWASE, K., HARA, K., and MIYAZ AKI, S. (1981) Long-term prognosis after infantile spasms: A statistical study of prognostic factors in 200 cases. *Dev. Med. Child Neurol.*, **23**, 51-65.

PAPINI, M., PASQUINELLI, A., ARMELLINI, M., and ORLANDI, D. (1984) Alertness and incidence of seizures in patients with Lennox-Gastaut syndrome. *Epilepsia*, **25**, 161-167.

PAVONE, L., INCORPORA, G., LA ROSA, M., LI VOLTI, S., and MOLLICA, F. (1981) Treatment of infantile spasms with sodium dipropylacetic acid. *Dev. Med. Child Neurol.*, **23**, 454-461.

RUKONEN, R., and DONNER, M. (1979) Incidence and aetiology of infantile spasms from 1960-1976: A population study in Finland. *Dev. Med. Child Neurol.*, **21**, 333-343.

SOREL, L., and DUSAUCY-BAULOYE, A. (1958) A propos de 21 cas d'hypsarhythmie Gibbs: Son traitement spectaculaire par l'ACTH. *Acta Neurol. Belg.*, **58**, 130-141.

SCHNEIDER, H., VASSELLA, F., and KARBOWSKI, K. (1970) The Lennox syndrome. A clinical study of 40 children. *Eur. Neurol.*, **4**, 289-300.

WATANABE, K., IWASE, K., and HARA, K. (1973) The evolution of EEG features in infantile spasms. *Dev. Med. Child Neurol.*, **15**, 584-596.

YAMATOGI, Y., OHTSUKA, Y., ISHIDA, T., ICHIBA, N., ISHIDA, S., MIYAKE, S., OKA, E., and OHTAHARA, S. (1979) Treatment of the Lennox syndrome with ACTH. A clinical and electroencephalographic study. *Brain Dev.*, **4**, 267-276.

ZELLWEGER, H. (1948) Krämpfe im Kindesalter. *Helv. Paediatr. Acta*, **3** (Suppl.), issue 5.

Paediatric Perspectives on Epilepsy
Edited by E. Ross and E. Reynolds
© 1985 John Wiley & Sons Ltd.

5

Fits and neurodegenerative disease

RICHARD ROBINSON
Newcomen Centre, Guy's Hospital, London

SUMMARY

Children with certain neurodegenerative conditions are known to be prone to epilepsy, though by no means all actually develop seizures. The proportion that do so appears to depend on the type and severity of the neurodegenerative changes and on the age of the child, i.e. the stage of brain maturation, which may also influence the seizure type. Although it is often stated that epilepsy is more characteristic of degenerative changes principally affecting the grey matter, rather than the white matter, a more detailed appraisal shows that the distinction is not clear-cut. Seizures occur in both types of condition, perhaps because degenerative changes are seldom confined to grey or white matter. However, neuronal histology shows no definite correlation with development of seizures. Dementia on the other hand is almost invariable (though not necessarily concurrent) in children with neurodegenerative disorders who develop seizures. It is difficult to formulate predictive correlates at present, but further studies could shed light on the multifactorial aetiology of epilepsy.

INTRODUCTION

Conditions primarily affecting grey matter are often said to be characterized by the early onset of fits and dementia, in contradistinction to white-matter disorders which are said to be typified by the evolution of long-tract signs in which seizures are not a prominent feature. How far these assumptions are justified is examined below, mainly by reference to three types of neurodegenerative condition, the leucodystrophies, the gangliosidoses and Batten's disease. They are also considered to see whether any other broad conclusions can be reached about the relationship between degenerative changes and liability to seizures. Although several conditions of unknown aetiology are covered, degenerative disorders caused by chronic infections and amino-acidopathies have been excluded.

LEUCODYSTROPHIES

There are several types of leucodystrophy, in all of which the white matter shows strikingly low attenuation on computer tomography. A good account of the group of metachromatic leucodystrophies reviews the findings in 38 cases (MacFaul *et al.*, 1982). Twenty-four of these children had the commonest late infantile form, which typically presents with deterioration of walking between the ages of six months and two years. Although spike-wave complexes were not commonly seen in their EEGs, six of these children, i.e. one-quarter, had fits which usually appeared within one year of the onset of symptoms. A further six children had juvenile-onset metachromatic leucodystrophy, which presented with educational and behavioural problems between the ages of six and 10 years. Four of these children, i.e. two-thirds, had fits which came on between two and four years after the onset of symptoms. Finally, MacFaul *et al.* proposed a new group, which they called 'early juvenile', presenting simultaneously with gait disorder and educational/behavioural problems between four and six years of age. In this group three out of seven had fits. In all, 13 out of the total group of 37 followed up had fits. This comparatively high incidence of fits in a disorder where they have been thought to be atypical is not altogether surprising, for although the hallmark of the histology is demyelination, sulphatide-containing intracellular material is found in groups of neurones both in the cerebral cortex and in subcortical structures.

By contrast, in the rarer leucodystrophy known as Krabbe's disease, seizures are distinctly uncommon. In this disorder, the cytoplasmic inclusions are found in globoid cells – which appear to be modified macrophages rather than neurones. Neuronal histology is characterized by cell loss rather than by survival with intracellular storage of abnormal material. This distinction is examined in more detail below.

A commoner form of leucodystrophy is adreno-leucodystrophy, in which fits may occur as the disease progresses – although here again the brunt of pathology falls on the white matter.

Two other conditions commonly included in the leucodystrophic group are the spongy degenerations of Canavan's disease and Alexander's disease. Although the spongiform changes characteristic of these diseases are most marked in the white matter and the histology is characterized by loss, rather than modification, of neurones, seizures are a feature of both conditions.

This brief survey of the leucodystrophies serves to demonstrate that: (1) seizures are relatively common; (2) there appears to be no close correlation, within the white matter disorders, between the neuronal histology seen on light microscopy and frequency of fits. Since not all areas of the brain are similarly epileptogenic, it may be worth examining the numbers and distribution of affected neurones in more detail. The gangliosidoses can serve as models.

GANGLIOSIDOSES

Fits are a characteristic feature of Tay–Sachs disease (Gm_2 gangliosidosis). It is possible that the exaggerated startle reaction typical of this condition is a form of stimulus-induced myoclonus. Gelastic attacks occur in addition, sometimes in association with frank seizures and sometimes independently. Seizures do not occur in the late-onset cases of this disorder, however, which present with ataxia and combined upper and lower motor neurone lesions simulating Friedrich's ataxia. Yet the central nervous system histology appears to be identical in both the early- and the late-onset forms, with lamellar cytoplasmic inclusions seen in nerve cells.

The same sort of variability is found in Farber's disease. Here, ceramide is deposited within neurones and around periarticular tissues, evoking an inflammatory response. In the handful of published cases, two had infantile spasms but the remainder were seizure free. However, in one unpublished case (Neville, personal communication), severe fits were a prominent feature from an early age.

In Gm_1 gangliosidosis, which usually presents at birth with coarse facial features, hepatosplenomegaly, kyphosis and delayed development, the storage material is also found in neurones. However only some, by no means all, patients so affected have fits.

Although not one of the gangliosidoses, neuro-axonal dystrophy shows the same discrepancy between histology and clinical characteristics. This autosomal-recessive condition is characterized by the slowing of motor development between six months and two years, with the development of pyramidal tract signs, notably hypotonia, and early visual involvement. The confirmatory histological finding consists of spheroid bodies in axonal endings in the cerebral cortex. Seizures are rare in the infantile variety of neuro-axonal dystrophy, but common in the infrequent juvenile-onset cases, although the histology is identical.

Within these conditions, therefore, the distribution of neuronal involvement does not appear to correlate with the presence of fits.

An alternative approach is to examine the temporal relationship between the evolution of symptoms and differential involvement within the nervous system. For example, are grey-matter disorders more likely to *present* with fits than white-matter disorders? The picture in children with spongy degeneration of the grey matter appears to support this idea. Although the characteristic microcystic degeneration of the grey matter is found in a great many metabolic disorders, the same changes are found in some children with no recognized metabolic error. A number of these are familial. Others, associated with liver impairment, earn the eponym of Huttenlocher's syndrome.

BATTEN'S DISEASE

The group of disorders known as Batten's disease can also shed some light on this question. Presenting clinically with amblyopia and dementia, these conditions have characteristic inclusions in the cytoplasm of cortical neurones. In the commonest late-infantile form, in which dementia precedes amblyopia, a variety of seizure types occurs, starting an average of eight months after the onset of symptoms. Myoclonic jerks may become continuous and very difficult to control. In the juvenile form, in which amblyopia precedes dementia, both major and minor seizures are a feature, starting at a mean interval of three years after the onset of symptoms. They may also become intractable. Finally (and least common in Britain), there is the infantile form which starts between eight and 18 months of age with concurrent dementia and visual failure. Typical myoclonic jerks are usually seen about one year after onset; they may be very complex, mimicking knitting movements. In none of these conditions, in which cortical neurones are primarily affected, are fits invariably an early feature.

OTHER NEURODEGENERATIVE CONDITIONS

It should be noted that a variety of seizure types occur in most of the conditions mentioned so far. Occasionally, however, the fits may be relatively stereotyped within a condition. In type C Niemann-Pick disease for instance, which is characterized by hepatosplenomegaly and vertical supranuclear ophthalmoplegia, when fits occur they are nearly always major motor ones. By contrast, in sialidosis 1, the cherry-red spot myoclonus syndrome which typically presents in adolescence with severe myoclonus and insidious visual loss, the fits are confined to myoclonus, as the name suggests.

As mentioned above, one might be tempted to suppose that dementia associated with alteration of neuronal activity (by, for example, storage material) would be more likely to cause fits than would dementia associated with neuronal loss. Although a condition such as Krabbe's disease appears to support this argument, seizures are a frequent and typical feature in conditions characterized by cortical neuronal loss, such as the grey-matter spongy degenerations, as well as conditions characterized by abnormal storage within neurones.

A notable discrepancy is that in the mucopolysaccharidosis group as a whole and in mannosidosis, which are all characterized by dementia and storage of abnormal material in cortical neurones, fits are infrequent and develop late in the course of the disease, if at all.

CONCLUSIONS

One rule which seems to emerge from this material is that in those neurodegenerative disorders where seizures occur, dementia is almost invariable although by no means concurrent. In 'Lafora body' disease, for example, myoclonus is an early feature, usually presenting between the ages of seven and 10 years, with intellectual deterioration as a subsequent event. I have seen one family with this condition in which a presymptomatic EEG showed multifocal spike-wave complexes in a child who subsequently developed the typical course with overt fits. One interesting feature of this condition is that the somatosensory evoked responses are greatly amplified, analogous to the amplified visual evoked responses typical of late infantile Batten's disease.

Whilst it is difficult to frame any convincing predictive correlates between seizures and neurodegenerative disorders, it is clear that there is sufficient discrepancy both within and between groups to suggest that they are useful models which may repay closer study of the aetiology of seizure disorders. Perhaps part of the answer will be found by adopting the multifactorial approach implied by Professor O'Donohoe's discussion (page 6) of the interplay between genetic susceptibilities and other variables, of which a storage disorder may be one.

REFERENCE

MacFaul, R., Cavanagh, N., Lake, B. D., Stephens, R., and Whitfield, A. E. (1982) Metachromatic leucodystrophy: Review of 38 cases. *Arch. Dis. Child.*, **57**, 168–175.

Paediatric Perspectives on Epilepsy
Edited by E. Ross and E. Reynolds
© 1985 John Wiley & Sons Ltd.

6

Seizures and mental handicap in the post-neonatal portion of the first year of life

GWILYM HOSKING

The Ryegate Centre, Children's Hospital, Sheffield

SUMMARY

Widespread damage to the brain can be manifested in a number of different ways. Its sequelae in the young child may include severe mental retardation, cerebral palsy and seizure disorders. It is rational therefore, when seizures are coupled with intellectual impairment, to suspect a structural basis in the brain and/or a biochemical cause for both conditions. The likelihood of seizures generally rises with the severity of intellectual impairment. In children with Down's syndrome, however, seizures are relatively infrequent, although intellectual impairment is common. If they do occur in Down's syndrome, management tends to be easier than in mental retardation due to other causes.

Aetiological factors linked to seizures in the first year of life are mainly pre- or perinatal, and over half the affected children have other problems, including cerebral palsy. Liability to seizures continues to be associated with intellectual impairment during childhood and adolescence. The cause should always be sought because not all cases are progressive and some may be remediable.

INTRODUCTION

The long-term sequelae of brain damage may include severe intellectual impairment, cerebral palsy and a seizure disorder (Hagberg and Kyllerman, 1983). This review considers those situations in the post-neonatal period of the first year of life where seizures occur in infants with probable intellectual impairment – concentrating on those in which the underlying disorder or dysfunction is assumed to be static, rather than inherently progressive.

At this period in an infant's life the epileptic threshold is believed to be relatively high, so that the occurrence of seizures at this time, in the absence of a simple remediable cause, may itself be an indication of widespread and severe underlying brain dysfunction. However, it is not always possible during the first year of life to determine whether an intellectual deficit is present or not. We shall therefore concentrate on those situations in which there is known to be at least a strong association between seizures and intellectual impairment, notably:

Chromosomal disorders;
Hydrocephalus;
Varied (other) structural abnormalities of the brain;
Neurocutaneous syndromes;
Cerebral palsy.

CHROMOSOMAL DISORDERS

Down's syndrome by itself accounts for the bulk of the major chromosomal abnormalities associated with severe (in most cases) intellectual impairment. It is almost always diagnosed readily at birth.

Seizures are frequently stated to be relatively uncommon in children and adults with Down's syndrome. This is almost certainly the case when comparisons are made with groups of patients with similar degrees of intellectual deficit but of different or unknown aetiologies. The exact incidence of seizures in Down's syndrome seems difficult to determine, with estimates varying from less than 1% to 10%. Veall (1974) gave a figure of 1.9% for a group under the age of 20 years, but in that study only a very small number was under the age of five years.

Over a period of five years in Sheffield we have seen a number of Down's syndrome infants with infantile spasms. The association between the two is not a new observation (Pollack *et al.*, 1978). The frequency figures based on data from our case register suggest that approximately 3.5% of children with Down's syndrome have infantile spasms. This figure is somewhat higher than the 2% given by Stephenson for the incidence of infantile spasms in Down's syndrome (unpublished data). Whatever figure may be accepted, it is useful to bear in mind that the incidence of infantile spasms is generally of the order of 0.02%. Although this may not be universally agreed, the onset of infantile spasms in Down's syndrome does not appear to bode well for that infant's subsequent development, compared with Down's infants in general. Nevertheless, the actual management of the infantile spasms has been relatively straightforward in our experience, and the development of ongoing seizures has been less frequent than expected.

Quite why this undoubted association between epilepsy and impaired development should exist in Down's syndrome remains speculative. It could, of course, quite simply reflect the underlying brain dysfunction that produces the inevitable intellectual impairments of Down's syndrome; other possibilities include hypoplasia of the cerebellum, an abnormality of serotonin metabolism, or an immunological disorder.

While Down's syndrome dominates the field of chromosome disorders, we have seen quite a large number of children with seizure disorders in whom we have found other chromosomal abnormalities. None of these has, however, been in a high enough number to allow even a guess at the frequency of a seizure disorder.

HYDROCEPHALUS

A retrospective study of 200 children with hydrocephalus (Hosking, 1974) showed the overall incidence of seizures to be approximately 30%. The incidence in those whose hydrocephalus was associated with a spina bifida lesion was 26%, and in those with post-meningitic hydrocephalus it was 54%. Among the former, 15% had the onset of their seizures within the first year of life, compared with 23% in the latter. Of the several factors considered, apart from the aetiology of the hydrocephalus itself, valve insertion appeared to bear a direct relationship to the occurrence of seizures. This inference was drawn from the observation that the incidence of seizure disorder rose with the number of valve revisions.

Ines and Markland (1977) found a seizure incidence of 18.2% in non-shunted patients and 65.4% in those with CSF shunts. Their EEG studies, and the focal nature of the attacks reported, all pointed to the proximal catheter of the shunt system as being a major cause for the seizures. These and similar findings have prompted many to recommend that the proximal catheter should, as far as possible, be inserted through an area of the lowest possible epileptogenicity.

OTHER STRUCTURAL ABNORMALITIES OF THE BRAIN

The relationship between seizures, severe intellectual impairment and gross brain malfunctions can be seen most dramatically in Aicardi's syndrome (Aicardi et al., 1969). This non-familial syndrome that occurs in girls comprises choroidal lacunae, intraventricular heteropias and callosal agenesis as well as vertebro-costal anomalies; it is invariably associated with infantile spasms and severe mental retardation.

Apart from Aicardi's syndrome, it has been our experience that, among children with an intellectual deficit associated with seizures, CT scanning reveals a high incidence of varied structural abnormalities – many of them midline.

NEUROCUTANEOUS SYNDROMES

Recognition in early infancy of some of the neurocutaneous syndromes may at times be straightforward, as it is in most but not all cases of the

Sturge–Weber syndrome. With other types, this may produce difficulties. Von Recklinghausen's disease, with its various associations, including intellectual deficit and seizure disorder, may be exceedingly difficult to recognize in early infancy. Tuberous sclerosis is more important in this context since the association of intellectual deficit and epilepsy is very strong. Classical adenoma sebaceum is a later and not invariable feature. A search for other cutaneous stigmata may prove difficult, though easier in more pigmented than in pale skin. Small areas of depigmentation of hair have been suggested by some as possibly the only cutaneous diagnostic clue from time to time. The importance of recognizing tuberous sclerosis does not need to be emphasized, and CT scanning should be mandatory. Skull radiology alone cannot be expected to help.

CEREBRAL PALSY

There is, of course, a close relationship between cerebral palsy, intellectual deficits, and epilepsy (Hagberg and Kyllerman, 1983). The incidence of severe intellectual impairment and epilepsy in the cerebral-palsied population as a whole is difficult to be certain about, with figures for epilepsy ranging between 30 and 58%. But in those with both cerebral palsy and a seizure disorder, together with a possible intellectual deficit, the overwhelming majority will be within the group of spastic cerebral palsies – hemiplegic and quadriplegic.

CONCLUSIONS

It is important to remind ourselves that, while figures may vary from one study to another, the overall incidence of seizures in the intellectually-impaired population is high. Richardson *et al.* (1980) reported a 27% seizure rate in a cohort of such persons aged 22, and an 11% rate in those considered 'borderline' intellectually impaired. From this cohort they were able to conclude, as others have (e.g. Corbett *et al.*, 1975), that the more severe the intellectual impairment, the stronger was the association with seizures, the more complex their nature, and the earlier their onset. Among these intellectually-impaired subjects with epilepsy, 12% had the onset of their seizures within the first year of life.

The interrelationship between major developmental deficits and seizures in the first year of life has been examined more recently by Matsumoto *et al.* (1982) in their studies of aetiological factors and the long-term prognosis for seizures within the first year of life. Their findings suggested that, in 40% of infants with seizures during the first year of life, the identifiable aetiological factors were prenatal and perinatal. Follow-up of those whose aetiology appeared to be prenatal revealed that 66% had other major development anomalies, compared with 55% among those whose aetiology appeared to be perinatal.

It is important in the infant with a seizure disorder of early onset to consider not only a structural basis for the combination of seizure disorder and intellectual impairment, but also the possibility of a biochemical cause. Such disorders do not always present in the neonatal period, and not all are inherently progressive.

REFERENCES

AICARDI, J., CHEVRIE, J. J., and ROUSSELIE, F. (1969) Le syndrome spasmes en flexion, agénésie calleuse, anomalies choriorétiniennes. *Arch. Fr. Pediatr.*, **26**, 1103-1120.

CORBETT, J. A., HARRIS, R., and ROBINSON, R. G. (1975) Epilepsy. In: *Mental Retardation and Developmental Disabilities*, **III**, pp. 81-111 (Ed. J. Wortis). Brunner, Mazel, New York.

HAGBERG, B., and KYLLERMAN, M. (1983) Epidemiology of mental retardation – a Swedish survey. *Brain Dev.*, **5**, 441-449.

HOSKING, G. P. (1974) Fits in hydrocephalic children. *Arch. Dis. Child.*, **49**, 633-635.

INES, D. F., and MARKLAND, O. N. (1977) Epileptic seizures and electro-encephalographic findings in hydrocephalus and their relation to shunting procedures. *Electroencephalog. Clin. Neurophysiol.*, **42**, 761-768.

LAGOS, J. C., and GOMEZ, M. R. (1967) Tuberous sclerosis: reappraisal of a clinical entity. *Mayo Clin. Proc.*, **42**, 26-49.

MATSUMOTO, A., WATANABE, K., SUGIURA, M., NEGORA, T., TAKAESU, E., and IWASE, K. (1982) Etiologic factors and long-term prognosis of convulsive disorders in the first year of life. *Neuropaediatrie*, **14**, 231-234.

POLLACK, M. A., GOLDEN, G. S., SCHMIDT, R., DAVIES, J. A., and LEEDS, N. (1978) Infantile spasms in Down's syndrome: A report of 5 cases and review of the literature. *Ann. Neurol.*, **3**, 406-408.

RICHARDSON, S. A., KOLLER, H., KATZ, M., and McLAREN, J. (1980) Seizures and epilepsy in a mentally retarded population over the first 22 years of life. *Appl. Res. Ment. Retard.*, **1**, 123-138.

VEALL, R. M. (1974) The prevalence of epilepsy among mongols, related to age. *J. Ment. Defic. Res.*, **18**, 99-106.

Paediatric Perspectives on Epilepsy
Edited by E. Ross and E. Reynolds
© 1985 John Wiley & Sons Ltd.

7

Pertussis immunization and fits

MARTIN H. BELLMAN[1] and EUAN M. ROSS[2]
[1]*Royal National Throat, Nose and Ear Hospital, London, and*
[2]*Paediatric Department, Charing Cross Hospital, London*

SUMMARY

Clustering of convulsions and other neurological reactions within a short time of pertussis immunization first suggested a causal association. Many types of neurological illness start in the first year of life, however, and pertussis vaccine is offered three times to infants in this age group. These events are therefore bound to occur in close time relation. When the 'normal' risk of seizures (10–17 per 1000 children aged 3–15 months) is broken down to give a daily expected range, this encompasses most of the published figures for the risk of convulsions after pertussis immunization. Thus, giving pertussis vaccine appears to add little to the numerical chances of developing a convulsive disorder. In addition, no clinical or pathological features characterize the convulsions or other neurological disorders that follow immunization. It is therefore likely that many of these conditions follow pertussis immunization by chance.

INTRODUCTION

Since 1933 there have been at least 47 published reports of neurological 'reactions' to pertussis vaccine. The vast majority (83%) of the total of 642 collected cases suffered convulsions; the remainder fell into three main groups: hemiplegia (7%), coma (6%), and sudden death (3%) (Bellman, 1984). The interval between immunization and onset of illness was recorded in 298 cases: in 75% it was less than 24 hours, with a further 11% in the subsequent 48 hours. It was this apparent clustering of reactions within a short time (three days) of immunization that led to the suggestion of a causal association between pertussis vaccine and neurological disorders. However, events occurring shortly after immunization attract particular attention and are more likely to be reported; no account was taken of chance association.

LEVEL OF RISK

Many types of neurological illness, with diverse causes, present during the first year of life. There is therefore a high chance of a close temporal association with immunization, which is offered to infants three times during this period. Tunstall-Pedoe and Rose (1981) reviewed the extant literature on childhood convulsions and concluded that the incidence of first convulsions for the age group 3–15 months (the age range in which the primary immunization course is given) was 10–17 per 1000 children per year. Their calculation of day-by-day risks gave a range which encompassed the risk figures suggested by several authors for convulsions after pertussis vaccine (Table I). The only figure outside this 'natural' risk range was from West Germany (Ehrengut, 1974), where the denominator of immunizations given may have been underestimated, thus exaggerating the risk figure.

Table I   Risk of convulsions during the first 24 hours and the first three days after pertussis immunization

	1 day	3 days
'Natural' risk		
	1 in 38 000	1 in 12 667
Tunstall-Pedoe and Rose, 1981	to	to
	1 in 20 000	1 in 6667
Pertussis vaccine risk		
		1 in 7347
MRC trials, 1956 and 1959		to
		1 in 11 835
Strom, 1967	1 in 23 000	
Hannik and Cohen, 1979		1 in 8100
Ehrengut, 1974	1 in 11 250	

Neurological reactions to immunization in Great Britain have been recorded as part of the National Childhood Encephalopathy Study (NCES) (Miller *et al.*, 1981). This epidemiological investigation identified the attributable risk (AR) of severe acute encephalopathy within seven days of pertussis immunization in all children, excluding infantile spasms, as 1 in 140 000. The AR of those illnesses in children who died or in whom there were persistent neuro-developmental sequelae was 1 in 330 000 immunizations when the child showed no neurological deficit before onset. The diagnostic spectrum of the notified encephalopathies varied widely (Table II). Statistical analysis showed no significant association with cases of infantile spasms, but suggested that pertussis immunization may act as a non-specific trigger for the onset of symptoms in children who were already predisposed to the development of spasms (Bellman *et al.*, 1983).

Table II   Diagnostic categories notified to the NCES

Diagnosis	Previously normal	Patients initially affected	Normal one year later Patients	(%)
Febrile convulsions*	337	372	311	(92)
Encephalitis/encephalopathy	305	344	150	(49)
Infantile spasms	156	268	52	(33)
Non-febrile convulsions*/ epilepsy	89	149	48	(54)
Reye's syndrome	47	49	10	(21)
Total	934	1182	571	(61)

* Duration >30 min or persistent neurological abnormality.

DIAGNOSTIC CATEGORIES

Case-control analysis with respect to combined diphtheria/tetanus/pertussis (DTP) immunization of previously normal children, regardless of outcome, is shown in Table III, according to diagnostic group. The greatest contributions to the relative risk (RR) of 2.87 for all diagnoses came from cases of convulsions (RR = 2.97) and of encephalitis/encephalopathy (RR = 3.74). The distinction

Table III   Case-control comparisons within seven days of DTP immunization in previously normal children – all outcomes

Diagnostic category		Immunized Children	(%)	Non-immunized Children	(%)	Relative risk (probability)
All diagnoses	Cases	34	(3.7)	889	(96.3)	2.87
	Controls	28	(1.5)	1791	(98.5)	($P<0.001$)
Infantile spasms	Cases	8	(5.2)	145	(94.8)	2.46
	Controls	7	(2.3)	294	(97.7)	(n.s.)
Encephalitis/ encephalopathy	Cases	11	(3.4)	311	(96.6)	3.74
	Controls	8	(1.3)	629	(98.7)	($P<0.025$)
Convulsions	Cases	14	(3.3)	407	(96.7)	2.97
	Controls	10	(1.2)	819	(98.8)	($P<0.01$)

between these two diagnostic categories was sometimes blurred, and the majority of children classified as encephalitis/encephalopathy had convulsions. Of the 426 cases classified as convulsions, 337 (79%) were diagnosed as febrile convulsions and 89 (21%) as non-febrile convulsions or epilepsy. There was again some diagnostic blurring of these two entities, as the definition of fever in the febrile convulsion cases was not consistent. The clinical features, however, tended to follow the patterns usually associated with these separate types of convulsion (Bellman, 1984). All cases in the NCES were followed up for one year after their initial neurological illness, using standard assessment procedures. Of the febrile convulsion cases, 92% appeared normal, whereas only 54% of the non-febrile convulsion cases were normal.

A case-control analysis for pertussis immunization in previously normal children who were abnormal on follow-up is shown in Table IV. Only one previously normal case diagnosed as 'convulsions' had persistent neurodevelopmental sequelae, so no relative risk could be calculated. In contrast,

Table IV Case-control comparisons within seven days of DTP immunization in previously normal children who were abnormal on follow-up

Diagnostic category		Immunized Children	(%)	Non-immunized Children	(%)	Relative risk (probability)
All diagnoses	Cases	11	(3.2)	332	(96.8)	2.75
	Controls	8	(1.2)	673	(98.8)	($P<0.05$)
Infantile spasms	Cases	4	(3.9)	98	(96.1)	1.60
	Controls	5	(2.5)	198	(97.5)	(n.s.)
Encephalitis/ encephalopathy	Cases	5	(3.5)	166	(96.5)	5.14
	Controls	2	(0.6)	341	(99.4)	($P<0.05$)
Convulsions	Cases	1	(1.9)	52	(98.1)	—
	Controls	0	(0.0)	106	(100)	—

the group shown in Table III included 14 children diagnosed as 'convulsions' who had received pertussis vaccine less than seven days previously, but whose outcome was not necessarily abnormal. It can be concluded therefore that convulsion cases contributed significantly to the overall risk of encephalopathy after pertussis immunization, regardless of outcome, but that they were virtually excluded from the risk of encephalopathy followed by persistent neurodevelopmental sequelae. Although febrile and non-febrile convulsions were not distinguished for the purposes of the case-control analyses, the individual diagnoses of the vaccine-associated cases (Table V) show that the majority of the convulsions were febrile and that most recovered.

CONCLUSIONS

No clinical or pathological features were identified which distinguished the illness suffered by the vaccine-associated cases from the remaining majority who were

Table V Pertussis-vaccine-associated cases (within seven days)

Diagnosis	Previously normal	Number	Development normal one year later
Febrile convulsions	12	14	12
Non-febrile convulsions/ epilepsy	2	4	1
Encephalitis/encephalopathy	11	11	6
Infantile spasms	8	9	4
Reye's syndrome	1	1	0
Total	34	39	23

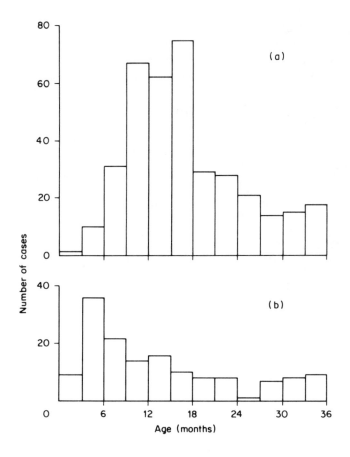

Fig. 1 The age distribution of (a) febrile and (b) non-febrile convulsions recorded in the National Childhood Encephalopathy Study

not vaccine associated. The relatively benign pattern of the illness and the age distribution (Fig. 1) of the febrile convulsions were similar to those usually associated with this disorder. Whatever the pathogenesis (possibly neurotoxic) of rare cases of severe encephalopathy time-associated with pertussis vaccine, it is likely that many convulsions have only a coincidental association with immunization. A feverish reaction to the vaccine is common and this may be the first non-specific triggering factor for a convulsion in a susceptible child. In these cases the ensuing neurological illness, which may have occurred during pyrexia due to other causes, should not be blamed directly on the vaccine.

ACKNOWLEDGEMENTS

The authors wish to thank their many co-workers on the National Childhood Encephalopathy Study, conducted initially at the Middlesex and subsequently at St Mary's Hospital Medical Schools, London, and in particular the co-director of the Study, Professor David Miller, and the statistician, Mrs Jane Wadsworth. The study was dependent on the goodwill of large numbers of parents, health visitors and doctors throughout the country, and was funded by the DHSS.

REFERENCES

BELLMAN, M. H. (1984) Serious acute neurological diseases of children. A clinical and epidemiological investigation with special reference to whooping cough disease and immunization. MD Thesis, University of London.

BELLMAN, M. H., ROSS, E. M., and MILLER, D. L. (1983) Infantile spasms and pertussis immunisation. *Lancet i*, 1031–1034.

EHRENGUT, W. (1974) Über convulsive Reaktionen nach Pertussis-schutzimpfung. *Dtsch. Med. Wochenschr.*, 99, 2273–2279.

HANNIK, C. A., and COHEN, H. (1979) Pertussis vaccine experience in the Netherlands. In: *International Symposium on Pertussis, Bethesda, 1978*, pp. 279–282 (Eds C. R. Manclark and J. C. Hill). US Department of Health, Education and Welfare, Washington DC.

MEDICAL RESEARCH COUNCIL (1956) Vaccination against whooping cough. Relation between protection in children and results of laboratory tests. *Br. Med. J.*, 2, 454–462.

MEDICAL RESEARCH COUNCIL (1959) Vaccination against whooping cough. *Br. Med. J.*, 1, 994–1000.

MILLER, D. L., ROSS, E. M., ALDERSLADE, R., BELLMAN, M. H., and RAWSON, N. S. B. (1981) Pertussis immunization and serious acute neurological illness in children. *Br. Med. J.*, 282, 1595–1599.

STROM, J. (1967) Further experience of reactions, especially of a cerebral nature, in conjunction with triple vaccination: a study based on vaccinations in Sweden, 1959–1965. *Br. Med. J.*, 4, 320–323.

TUNSTALL-PEDOE, H., and ROSE, G. (1981) Frequency and outcome of febrile and non-febrile convulsions in infancy. In: *Whooping Cough. Reports from the Committee on Safety of Medicines and the Joint Committee on Vaccination and Immunisation, DHSS*, pp. 50–54. HMSO, London.

Discussion

Dr J. A. Corbett (London): Could I ask Dr Hosking whether infantile spasms and myoclonic seizures in Down's syndrome ever respond to pyridoxine? When 5-hydroxy tryptophan was given in Down's syndrome to improve muscle tone, it produced myoclonic seizures; and there are animal models of myoclonic seizures associated with tryptophan abnormalities. Is there any evidence that myoclonic seizures later in childhood may respond to pyridoxine as one occasionally sees infantile spasms responding?

Hosking: I do not know of any validated studies on infantile spasms in Down's syndrome being treated with pyridoxine, although the issue has certainly been discussed.

Neville: Could Keith Brown tell us why he gives a trial dose of diazepam, rather than other benzodiazepines – and perhaps say something about the differences between them?

Brown: We use diazepam to test for benzodiazepine sensitivity mainly because we have seen severe bronchorrhoea from clonazepam. I do not know of any difference between the benzodiazepines in their inhibitory action on supposedly sensitized GABA receptors, which is thought to lessen the seizure discharge. However, the benzodiazepines may differ in the duration of their actions. Diazepam has a half-life of 15–20 minutes, and the anticonvulsant effect wears off thereafter, whereas the anxiolytic and muscle relaxant effects last very much longer. In other words, there seems to be a dissociation between anticonvulsant, hypnotic and anxiolytic effects – and this may be different for other benzodiazepines. Clinically patients habituate much more rapidly to clonazepam than to nitrazepam. We have therefore reverted to nitrazepam as our oral benzodiazepine. If we don't know whether to put the dosage up in a child with ongoing epileptic activity, we give another dose and monitor the EEG; if the activity disappears, we raise the dose. The presence of beta-activity has been suggested as evidence of a reasonable blood level, but many of these children don't get beta-activity, so we do not find this useful. The problem in children with the Lennox–Gastaut syndrome is to stop the fits *and* to keep them awake.

Dr M. J. Noronha (Manchester): Dr Brown raised the question of cytomegalovirus infection in West's syndrome and the dangers of giving ACTH. In the early 1970s I did a retrospective survey of 70 children with cytomegalovirus infection; 15% of them were abnormal but not one had had infantile spasms. Among children with infantile spasms that we have screened for virus infections, not one has had cytomegalovirus infection.

Brown: The Finnish survey suggested that cytomegalovirus infection was important, and deaths from activation of herpes viruses have been attributed to ACTH. There is evidence that cytomegalovirus, like any other herpes virus, can be activated by steroids. I accept that many children with infantile spasms do not excrete cytomegalovirus, but significant associations have been reported.

Dr S. H. Green (Birmingham): In the infantile spasm group of children, whether symptomatic or otherwise, do you think that the peculiar autistic-like behaviour or language deterioration is specifically a response to seizures or encephalopathy in the first year of life? Or is there something about the hypsarrhythmic type of picture which in some way interferes with language development? Occasionally, other seizures in the first year of life appear to be followed by language deterioration.

Ross: Infantile spasms comprise a far wider range of problems than we ever see in hospital neurology units. For example, a child may for a couple of days have infantile-spasm-like behaviour, which then goes away again. In one such case, I did three EEGs in a week, on Monday, Wednesday and Friday; only the Wednesday tracing was abnormal. We need to study the minor degrees of these conditions.

Brown: Spasms can occur with hypsarrhythmia or with a normal EEG. The spasms themselves do not seem to be related to brain damage or to the long-term prognosis; they sometimes affect an otherwise normal child. Hypsarrhythmia is not a specific EEG sign of an infantile spasm; it is an associated finding. But, just as the Lennox–Gastaut children appear to go into minor status, there may be unrecognized minor status in West's syndrome. It would be interesting to time the multifocal EEG spikes to see whether they coincide with the small focal myoclonic movements observed clinically. This could be a sort of epileptic polymyoclonia, in which non-verbal communication is lost, perhaps because of limbic spread. At this age, verbal communication has not yet developed.

Professor J. Aicardi (Paris): We have had extensive experience with infantile spasms, and I am not quite sure that spasms without hypsarrhythmia in a child with normal mentality is absolutely the same entity. I would not make a diagnosis of infantile spasms without at least some form of EEG abnormality.

Secondly, what proportion of patients with 'idiopathic' infantile spasms are cured in your experience? One cannot avoid being very much impressed by the fact that those patients who are indeed cured not only recover from the spasms but also have no residual mental disturbance. However, some of these patients, even when they become more or less normal intellectually later on, do keep rather bizarre behaviour, even in their twenties or later. One of my earliest patients is now an engineer in Paris and is quite intelligent but he is almost a schizophrenic. Many of them are like this, and I should like to have your comments.

Brown: As a group, mentally handicapped children with infantile spasms have a lot of communication and social interaction problems that you would not see in, say, a Down's child of similar IQ. This continues long term, and is not confined to the early stages.

I fully agree that when a child has a salaam attack, but is intellectually normal and has not got hypsarrhythmia, we should not diagnose infantile spasms. That is why I use the term West's syndrome because 'infantile spasm' is merely a description of the fit. Unless we group this together with hypsarrhythmia and ACTH responsiveness as West's syndrome, we shall have 20 different syndromes . . .

Dr B. D. Bower (Oxford): You said that the ketogenic diet was occasionally effective in Lennox–Gastaut. In our experience, if one of the three ketogenic diets available is applied properly and consistently, a better than 50% reduction in seizures can be achieved over a period of three months in 80% of Lennox–Gastaut cases. It is well worth trying and allows medication to be reduced or even withdrawn, so that the child is not walking around like a zombie from benzodiazepines.

Professor O. Eeg-Olofsson (Linköping, Sweden): Dr Brown, have you used cerebrospinal fluid analysis as a guide to therapy in infantile spasms and astatic myoclonic epilepsy? In my experience, oligoclonal banding on CSF electrophoresis is an indication to treat these children with steroids.

Brown: I have no experience. Would you tell us more about it?

Eeg-Olofsson: I have studied a few cases, especially those with astatic myoclonic or very therapy-resistant epilepsy who showed oligoclonal banding in their CSF. We have a method for demonstrating these bands on 5 microlitres of unconcentrated CSF. A girl with this finding who was very therapy resistant on ordinary anticonvulsants became completely seizure free after a couple of days on corticosteroids. She now has normal mental development, with generalized tonic-clonic seizures only about once or twice a year. She is on a small dose of carbamazepine at the moment. She was around two when she started to have those seizures, and is now six years old.

Dr C. R. Kennedy (Southampton): It is difficult to know how you could search for immunological abnormalities in children with pertussis-vaccine-related encephalopathies before it has been definitely decided whether the condition exists. However, a prospective study of 30 children who did have acute encephalopathy demonstrated virus infections in over 80%; they were all studied for immunological abnormalities, and none of them showed any evidence of deficiencies of cell-mediated or humoral immunity. What they did show was very high levels of immunoglobulin subclasses 1 and 3, but it is not yet possible to say whether these might reflect the fact that they had an active virus infection or some sort of hyper-responsive predisposition.

Dr S. M. Tucker (London): I am not convinced by the pertussis vaccine study, although I have read it repeatedly. What worries me is the incidence for encephalopathy in this country, given as one in 300 000, whereas the Americans quote a risk of one in 900 000. So the Americans licence the vaccine and say you cannot go to school without it. We do not do that here. The vaccines are obviously different, and I for one would not use the British vaccine. I have personally seen children who are perfectly well one day, have the vaccine, and are in considerable trouble that same evening. I am sure others must have had the same experience, but do not want to be quoted.

Ross: The British pertussis vaccine policy was established in the late 1950s, after the MRC compared about seven candidate vaccines (some of American origin) and selected one. There have been no direct, proper comparative studies between our vaccine and those produced in other countries. Among studies that have been done, surveys of acute side effects showed fewer British children developing fevers with our vaccines than American children given their vaccine. However, all this may very soon be history. New vaccines are rapidly on the way because the antigenic properties of the pertussis organism have been identified. Now, the need is for proper epidemiological studies of the new vaccines as they come along.

Tucker: The present British vaccine is also less effective than the American one.

Ross: Ours may be less protective, but the Americans give five injections in most states; we give three.

O'Donohoe: I do not like to use eponyms, much as I respect people like Henri Gastaut, and I would like to remind you what our distinguished visitor from France, Professor Aicardi, said as long as 11 years ago. He referred to these severe generalized epilepsies in young children as a heterogeneous group of disorders. They are certainly age related. An example is the newly-recognized Ohtahara syndrome – an eponym, I am afraid, for severe epileptic encephalopathy in the first month of life. Heterogeneity is to be seen in the fact that some children with infantile spasms do extremely well and recover, while the majority do not. Equally, not all generalized myoclonic epilepsies are bad; those occurring in three- and four-year-olds respond well to treatment, particularly with sodium valproate. Severe epilepsies occur in association with certain lesions, some of them related to serious infections, whereas others with strong hereditary influences respond better to treatment. I would not like you to go away with the idea that all myoclonic epilepsies do badly, but certainly those that begin in the first year of life do so – even the children who get febrile convulsions at that age tend to get them very severely. What this afternoon has highlighted is that we need to learn much more about why children develop these serious disorders in this particular age group. Perhaps we are on the brink of making some progress here.

Part III: Epilepsy in the pre-school child

Paediatric Perspectives on Epilepsy
Edited by E. Ross and E. Reynolds
© 1985 John Wiley & Sons Ltd.

8

Epileptic syndromes in childhood – overview and classification

JEAN AICARDI
Service Enfants Malades, Hôpital Necker, Paris

SUMMARY

The different clinical pictures of childhood epilepsy characteristic of particular age groups, and the fact that seizure patterns tend to evolve with age, demand a system of classification into epileptic syndromes. The relevant features include seizure type(s), mode of recurrence, neurological findings and the results of EEG and other investigations. Each epileptic syndrome may have several causes and/or outcomes. Some are quite specific and run a predictable course, while others are relatively loose associations, and a few remain unclassified because they do not constitute recognized syndromes. Individual classifications need to be revised as a child grows up. Not only do the causes and types of epilepsy differ according to the age of onset; the effects of seizures (brain damage; psychological and social sequelae), the EEG findings, the metabolism of anti-epileptic drugs and the prognosis also change with age.

INTRODUCTION

Epilepsy is much more common in infancy and childhood than at any other period of life. The epilepsies of childhood are also much more variable in expression and outcome than those of adults. In an individual child, the clinical and EEG features of epilepsy can change considerably with age. For example, partial seizures can precede infantile spasms which, in turn, may be followed by partial complex seizures or by the Lennox–Gastaut syndrome. Moreover, the clinical expression of seizures in young patients is often atypical as a result of incomplete development of synaptic and interhemispheral connections. Typical grand mal attacks are rare before two or three years of age, for instance,

65

and complex partial seizures at this age are manifested only by autonomic symptoms, loss of contact, and generalized hypo- or hypertonia.

As a result, classification should be limited to the delineation of *epileptic syndromes*, clusters of signs and symptoms occurring together. The features of such a syndrome may be clinical (seizure type(s), mode of seizure recurrence, neurological findings) or the results of EEG or other special investigations. A syndrome may have several causes and/or outcomes. Some are relatively specific, with a predictable course (e.g. benign rolandic epilepsy). Others are rather loose associations which do not permit an exact prediction of prognosis or help in deciding ·whether complementary investigations are necessary (e.g. partial complex seizures). A number of epilepsies do not constitute syndromes and therefore remain unclassified (e.g. many epilepsies with grand mal seizures, and epilepsies of young infants).

Epileptic syndromes are not the same in children of different ages. In addition, the effects of seizures (brain damage, and psychological and social changes) vary with the age of the patient – as do the causes of epilepsy, the metabolism of anti-epileptic drugs and the prognosis. Four main periods can be defined (Table I). This paper is mainly concerned with the third period and part of the second (covering the age range from one to nine years), and deals exclusively with chronic seizure disorders, not occasional and/or provoked seizures.

THREE MONTHS TO THREE OR FOUR YEARS

Epileptic syndromes in this age group are characterized by the rarity of typical grand mal seizures which is probably due to incomplete maturation of interhemispheral pathways. However, massive myoclonus and generalized tonic seizures are among the main seizure types in this period. Partial seizures (especially complex partial seizures) usually have a relatively limited expression. On the EEG, rapid spike-wave complexes (> 2.5 Hz) are uncommon and, when present, are of the irregular type. Rhythmic 3 Hz spike-wave discharges are not seen, but slow spike-waves at 1–2.5 Hz are a frequent EEG manifestation at this age. These slow spike-waves are often asymmetrical and may be asynchronous. Seizure discharges commonly consist of fast, low-voltage activity or of simple flattening of tracings. Brain damage of multiple causes is the predominant cause of epilepsy and the prognosis is, accordingly, guarded.

The main syndromes observed are shown in Table II. The early myoclonic epilepsies remain a somewhat controversial group. Isolated myoclonic attacks may have a relatively favourable outcome in comparison with the Lennox-Gastaut syndrome or with infantile spasms (Aircardi, 1980). Severe forms exist, however, and these are often associated with early prolonged, clonic seizures and with episodes of 'absence' status (Dravet et al., 1982).

Partial and generalized seizures in this age range are often impossible to classify (Chevrie and Aicardi, 1977). The outcome of such cases is difficult to

Table I The influence of age: the four main periods of childhood epilepsy and their main features

Period	Clinical features	Cerebral features and maturation
Neonatal (up to 2–3 months)	Lesional causes Fragmentary and erratic seizures No occasional seizures	Predominance of inhibitory influences Incomplete development of synapses and commissural connections High incidence of lesional brain damage
Second (3 months to 3–4 years)	Maximum incidence of occasional seizures Lesional causes still common Specific syndromes (e.g. West's and Lennox–Gastaut)	Predominance of excitatory influences Very high susceptibility of the brain to changes in homoeostasis Commissural connections still incompletely functional Rapid maturation of synaptic connections
Third (3–4 years to 9–10 years)	Rarity of occasional seizures Predominance of cryptogenic epilepsies (including partial cryptogenic epilepsies)	Relatively complete development of synaptic and interhemispheral connections Full development of system(s) responsible for synchronized paroxysmal activity (spike-wave) Lesser susceptibility to extraneural changes (hormonal)
Fourth (after 9–10 years)	Predominance of cryptogenic epilepsies (mainly primary generalized types)	

Table II　Main epileptic syndromes with onset in children aged 3
months to 3–4 years

Syndromes

Infantile spasms or West's syndrome (< 1 year)

Lennox–Gastaut syndrome (1–7 years)

Early myoclonic epilepsies (1–5 years)
— severe
— relatively benign

Epilepsies with partial seizures (of lesional origin)

Epilepsies with generalized seizures

Features

High incidence

Lesional origin in a majority of cases (< 2 years)

Frequent associations with neurological signs and/or mental
retardation

Outcome often unfavourable

Frequency of certain seizure types, including infantile spasms, tonic
seizures, myoclonic seizures, partial seizures (often with atypical
or limited expression; EEG patterns irregular)

EEG abnormalities mainly multifocal or partial; often ill-defined;
rarity of 3 Hz pattern; frequency of abnormal background

---

predict but is mainly severe (Cavazzuti *et al.*, 1984; Chevrie and Aicardi, 1978).
Generalized seizures without evidence of brain damage and a positive family
history of seizures have a better prognosis.

THREE TO 10 YEARS OF AGE

These syndromes are mainly of non-lesional origin and their prognosis
is consequently favourable. The full development of CNS pathways make
highly organized paroxysmal EEG activity possible, and this activity is often
rhythmic at 3 Hz. The main seizure types are typical grand mal seizures
and typical absences. A remarkable feature of this period is the occurrence
of epilepsies with partial seizures not related to localized brain damage (Aicardi,
1983). The main epileptic syndromes in this age range are displayed in
Table III.

Typical absence epilepsy (petit mal) is remarkable clinically and by its response
to certain drugs (ethosuximide). It is, however, a heterogeneous syndrome. Cases
with preceding or associated grand mal or intense myoclonic jerks have an
unfavourable outcome.

Table III   Main epileptic syndromes with onset in children aged 3–4
to 9–10 years

Syndromes

With generalized seizures

Grand mal following febrile convulsions

Other grand mal?

Typical absences (petit mal)

Late myoclonic epilepsies

With partial seizures

Benign epilepsy with centro-temporal foci

Benign epilepsy with occipital spike-wave

Other 'benign' partial epilepsies

Partial epilepsies of lesional origin (including HHE syndrome)

Features

Incidence lower than in younger children

Lesional causes decline in importance

Cryptogenic epilepsies with positive genetic factors

Infrequently associated with neurological signs and/or mental
retardation; outcome often favourable

Main seizure types include:
(1) Absences
(2) Generalized tonic-clonic seizures
(3) Several types of partial seizures with well-defined features

EEG abnormalities bilateral symmetric (often 3 Hz spike-wave
pattern) or focal and well defined

Benign epilepsy with centro-temporal spike foci is common and well individualized (Aicardi, 1983). Partial motor seizures characteristically affect the face and are related to sleep and repetitive central spike focus on a normal background rhythm. When the clinical and EEG features are typical, no radiological investigation is indicated and disappearance of seizures regularly occurs before adulthood. More recently, other types of 'benign' partial epilepsy have been described. Epilepsy with continuous occipital spike-waves arrested by eye opening (Gastaut, 1982) may be less benign than initially thought (Newton and Aicardi, 1983). Atypical partial benign epilepsy (Aicardi and Chevrie, 1982) should not be confused with the Lennox–Gastaut syndrome, despite the intense slow spike-wave activity and myo-atonic seizures seen in these patients. Its benignity, however, may be only relative. 'Benign' epilepsies with complex partial seizures (Dalla Bernardina *et al.*, 1980) and with evoked parietal spikes (De Marco and Tassinari, 1981) have been reported, but their nosological position is unclear at present.

Partial epilepsies of lesional origin are less common in this age range. The seizures are often complex partial in type and may follow prolonged unilateral seizures of early infancy (the hemiconvulsion–hemiplegia–epilepsy, or HHE, syndrome).

CHILDREN OVER NINE YEARS OF AGE

This period (which overlaps with the preceding one) is also characterized by the predominance of non-lesional epilepsies. Three main syndromes are common:

Epilepsy on awakening or nocturnal grand mal;
Massive conscious myoclonic jerks of the arms, generally upon awakening (benign juvenile myoclonic epilepsy – or Janz's syndrome) (Delgado-Escueta and Enrile-Bascal, 1984);
Typical absences, less frequently repeated than in younger patients.

These three syndromes often occur with various associations in the same patient. Partial seizures continue to occur in this period. Loiseau *et al.* (1983) have underlined the relative frequency in adolescents of isolated partial seizures (often occurring in a cluster).

CONCLUSION

The enormous variability of the types of epilepsy encountered in childhood make it imperative to study and describe the clinical features of the patients precisely and not just to classify them loosely into three or four groups. Precise assignment to well-defined syndromes will often permit much greater precision in prognosis and better management.

REFERENCES

AICARDI, J. (1980) Course and prognosis of certain childhood epilepsies with predominantly myoclonic attacks. In: *Advances in Epileptology. The XIth Epilepsy International Symposium*, pp. 159–163 (Eds J. A. Wada and J. K. Penry). Raven Press, New York.

AICARDI, J. (1983) The benign epilepsies of childhood. In: *Research Progress in Epilepsy*, pp. 231–239 (Ed. Rose F. Clifford). Pitman, London.

AICARDI, J., and CHEVRIE, J. J. (1982) Atypical benign partial epilepsy of childhood. *Dev. Med. Child Neurol.*, **24**, 281–292.

CAVAZZUTI, G. B., FERRARI, P., and LALLA, M. (1984) Follow-up study of 482 cases with convulsive disorders in the first year of life. *Dev. Med. Child Neurol.*, **26**, 425–437.

CHEVRIE, J. J., and AICARDI, J. (1977) Convulsive disorders in the first year of life: etiologic factors. *Epilepsia*, **18**, 489–498.

CHEVRIE, J. J., and AICARDI, J. (1978) Convulsive disorders in the first year of life: mortality, neurological and mental outcome. *Epilepsia*, **19**, 67–74.

DALLA BERNARDINA, B., BUREAU, M., DRAVET, C., DULAC, O., TASSINARI, C. A., and ROGER, J. (1980) Epilepsie bénigne de l'enfant avec crises de séméiologie affective. *Rev. EEG Neurophysiol.*, **10**, 8–18.

DELGADO-ESCUETA, A. V., and ENRILE-BASCAL, F. (1984) Juvenile myoclonic epilepsy of Janz. *Neurology (Cleveland)*, **34**, 285–294.

DE MARCO, P., and TASSINARI, C. A. (1981) Extreme somatosensory evoked potential (ESEP): an EEG sign forecasting the possible occurrence of seizures in children. *Epilepsia*, **22**, 569–575.

DRAVET, C., ROGER, J., BUREAU, M., and DALLA BERNARDINA, B. (1982) Myoclonic epilepsies in childhood. In: *Advances in Epileptology. The XIIIth Epilepsy International Symposium*, pp. 135–140 (Eds H. Akimoto, H. Kazamatsuri, M. Seino *et al.*). Raven Press, New York.

GASTAUT, H. (1982) A new type of epilepsy: benign partial epilepsy of childhood with occipital spike-waves. In: *Advances in Epileptology, The XIIIth Epilepsy International Symposium*, pp. 19–24 (Eds H. Akimoto, H. Kazamatsuri, M. Seino *et al.*). Raven Press, New York.

LOISEAU, P., DARTIGUES, J. F., and PESTRE, M. (1983) Prognosis of partial epileptic seizures in the adolescent. *Epilepsia*, **24**, 472–481.

NEWTON, R., and AICARDI, J. (1983) Clinical findings in children with occipital spike-wave complexes suppressed by eye-opening. *Neurology (Cleveland)*, **33**, 1526–1529.

Paediatric Perspectives on Epilepsy
Edited by E. Ross and E. Reynolds
© 1985 John Wiley & Sons Ltd.

9

Febrile convulsions

D. P. Addy
Dudley Road Hospital, Birmingham

SUMMARY

Febrile convulsions in children are uncommonly followed by the development
of other forms of seizure disorder. It is not possible to define a group of children
at very high risk of epilepsy within the 3% of all children who have febrile
convulsions. So-called 'atypical febrile convulsions' do not seem to differ as
regards pathogenesis in any essential respect from other febrile convulsions.
The definition of febrile convulsions should therefore be broad enough to
include prolonged or focal seizures. The risk of subsequent epilepsy is low,
at about 1.6%, compared with 0.5% for young children without febrile
convulsions. Three risk factors have been identified for the development of
epilepsy following febrile convulsions: family history of epilepsy in a first degree
relative, neurological abnormality after the first convulsion, and prolonged or
focal convulsions. Lumbar puncture need not be performed routinely in the
investigation of febrile convulsions, and continuous anticonvulsant therapy is
seldom indicated. There is no evidence that giving anticonvulsant drugs to
children with febrile convulsions prevents them from developing subsequent
epilepsy.

DEFINITION

Febrile convulsions are defined as: 'Convulsions with fever in children aged
between six months and five years without evidence of serious acute intracranial
disease or meningitis or of longstanding brain disease'. Convulsions associated
with infections that invade the central nervous system are therefore excluded. For
the purposes of research or professional discussion it is, however, counterproduc-
tive to exclude from the definition of febrile convulsions those children who have
prolonged or focal convulsions. In the 1950s a vogue arose for restricting

73

the term febrile convulsions to brief generalized seizures (Livingston, 1972; Friderichsen and Melchior, 1954; Prichard and McGreal, 1958). Livingston (1972) claimed that children with febrile convulsions could be divided into two groups: 'simple febrile convulsions' with a 3% risk of developing epilepsy, usually before the age of five years, and prolonged or focal seizures, classified as 'epilepsy precipitated by fever', where the risk of epilepsy was said to be 97%. No-one since that time has been able to define a group of children without structural lesions who have febrile convulsions followed by such a high chance of developing epilepsy.

PREVALENCE AND PROGNOSIS

A very different picture has emerged from the most complete study of febrile convulsions yet performed, the American National Collaborative Perinatal Project (Nelson and Ellenberg, 1976, 1978). Among approximately 54 000 babies followed from birth, 1706 developed febrile convulsions. Three risk factors for epilepsy were identified: family history of epilepsy in a first-degree relative, neurological abnormality after the first convulsions, and prolonged or focal convulsions. Children with two or three of these risk factors were found to have a 10% risk of epilepsy, compared with 1.6% for all children with febrile convulsions, and 0.5% for children who did not have febrile convulsions. Children with only one of the three risk factors had about the same rate for subsequent epilepsy (1.6%) as the whole febrile convulsion group. There was no evidence that prolonged or focal febrile convulsions differed fundamentally from brief generalized convulsions. As regards permanent sequelae, the American perinatal project showed the risk of death to be zero, and the risk of neurological damage to be very low. Although prolonged convulsions may cause brain lesions such as mesial temporal sclerosis, it is likely that most children who develop epilepsy after febrile convulsions already have a predisposition to epilepsy, whether genetic or structural, that is present before the first convulsion. The individual child with febrile convulsions has a very low risk of developing temporal lobe epilepsy although prolonged febrile convulsions are a common antecedent in people with chronic temporal lobe epilepsy subjected to temporal lobectomy.

PROPHYLAXIS

In deciding whether to give prolonged anticonvulsant therapy, a balance has to be drawn between the risk of neurological damage from recurrent seizures, if the child remains untreated, and the risks of drug toxicity. There is no evidence that giving anticonvulsant medication to children with febrile convulsions prevents their developing epilepsy (National Institutes of Health Consensus Development Panel, 1980). It is, however, very important to distinguish subsequent epilepsy from recurrent febrile convulsions, which are much more frequent but generally less serious. The overall risk of febrile convulsions recurring is about 30%, with the highest recurrence rates in the youngest age group. Indeed, febrile convulsions under the age of one year may be potentially more serious, calling for some caution in prognosis. As the age of the child at the time of the first convulsion rises, the likelihood of recurrence falls.

The main indication for continuous anticonvulsant therapy is the recurrence of febrile convulsions at a frequency which is intolerable to the parents. This especially applies to younger children. Only two drugs have been shown to be effective in reducing the number of recurrences, phenobarbitone and sodium valproate. Sodium valproate is probably the more effective of the two, but it also carries a greater risk of serious, even lethal, toxicity. Neither drug is satisfactory and, in my opinion, continuous prophylactic treatment should usually be avoided; but where it becomes necessary I prefer phenobarbitone because of the rare but potentially lethal hepatitis which may occur in the first 10 weeks of sodium valproate treatment (Addy, 1981). As always in paediatrics, the final decision on anticonvulsant therapy will depend on the wishes of the parents and their likely compliance. Increasingly I give the parents a supply of rectal diazepam, so that they are equipped for treating recurrent convulsions. They certainly find this helpful, even if they never actually give the drug.

ADMISSION TO HOSPITAL?

The proportion of children with febrile convulsions who are admitted to hospital has risen considerably, a fact demonstrated in Chapter 16 of this book. To a large extent this appears to be self-referral. An increasing proportion of parents have cars and prefer to get their children immediately to a hospital rather than wait for the family doctor to get to their home. As a result, convulsions are treated cearlier than in the past and this may be one of the reasons why the outcome for febrile convulsions appears to be better than it was. Although admission to hospital has potential disadvantages, in that the child is transferred to an alien environment, it does give the opportunity for close observation of the child. Admission to hospital may also protect the child from the early administration of antibiotics which can mask the development of meningitis or urinary tract infection. For these reasons many paediatricians encourage the admission of children with a febrile convulsion to hospital, particularly the first time it occurs. A study from Nottingham recently showed that about 70% of parents seeing their child having the first febrile convulsion thought that the child was going to die. This degree of alarm is often enough to warrant hospital admission but a general práctitioner may justifiably elect to manage a child at home if the child seems well after the convulsion, if the parents are sensible and able to cope, and if the general practitioner is prepared to keep a close eye on the child's progress. For those admitted to hospital after a first febrile convulsion there is no need for routine hospital follow-up. This is the province of the general practitioner, to whom the child can often be returned within 24 hours of the seizure.

ADVICE TO PARENTS

Few parents have any pre-existing knowledge about convulsions before the first one occurs in their child. For this reason they require a great deal of education both about the nature of febrile seizures and the fact that they rarely cause long-term brain damage. They need to know what to do when a fit occurs. Traditionally we teach parents to cool their children by removing clothes, sponging down with tepid water and giving cooling drinks and paracetamol (in preference to aspirin, which is no more effective and potentially more toxic). The success of these therapeutic measures, however, has never been properly assessed. There is some evidence that over-rapid cooling of the child may cause peripheral vasoconstriction and even raise the child's central core temperature. Probably the most useful measure is to teach parents about the importance of a rising temperature and prophylactic measures to be taken when their child seems hot. Few British parents own thermometers, in contrast to those across the Atlantic. There is still much dispute as to whether temperature taking should be encouraged or not. Rectal diazepam as Stesolid solution, which comes in handy plastic enema packs, is a useful step forward because the parents can then readily insert diazepam in a form that is rapidly absorbed. Although no conclusive British work has been done with this procedure it is certainly welcomed by the majority of parents, who are glad to have an effective measure that they can safely use.

INVESTIGATIONS

Routine biochemical tests and skull X-rays on children with febrile convulsions are an unnecessary and unjustified expense. The need for routine lumbar puncture to exclude meningitis has long been debated. Where there is clinical doubt a lumbar puncture should be performed but I do not believe that it is

Table I   Routine lumbar puncture after first febrile convulsion

	Number of lumbar punctures	Meningitis	
		Bacterial	Aseptic
Wolfe, 1978	309	0	0
Rollin and Masson, 1979	242	0	0
Heijbel et al., 1980	47	0	0
Rutter and Smales, 1977	314	1	3
Lorber and Sunderland, 1980	279	0	1

necessary in every case. In the Nottingham study, the CSF was normal in 310 out of the 314 children examined – and two of those with normal CSF developed meningitis. A normal finding can therefore be seriously misleading. Among the four children with abnormal CSF, three had viral meningitis, for which there is no specific therapy. The fourth had *Haemophilus influenzae* meningitis, but the clinical indications for lumbar puncture were unmistakable. In other words, lumbar puncture contributed little to the diagnosis. The findings of the Sheffield study of lumbar puncture in children with febrile convulsions point to similar convulsions (Table I). A reasonably experienced doctor pursuing a policy of close observation and lumbar puncture only when indicated by the clinical findings does not put his patients at increased risk (Lorber and Sunderland, 1980).

REFERENCES

ADDY, D. P. (1981) Prophylaxis and febrile convulsions. *Arch. Dis. Child.*, **56**, 81–83.

FRIDERICHSEN, C., and MELCHIOR, J. (1954) Febrile convulsions in children, their frequency and prognosis. *Acta Paediatr.* (Suppl. 100), **43**, 307–317.

HEIJBEL, J., BLOM, S., and BERGFORS, P. G. (1980) Simple febrile convulsions. A prospective incidence study and an evaluation of investigations initially needed. *Neuropaediatrie*, **11**, 45–56.

LIVINGSTON, S. (1972) *Comprehensive Management of Epilepsy in Infancy, Childhood and Adolescence*, pp. 16–33. Thomas, Springfield, Ill.

LORBER, J., and SUNDERLAND, R. (1980) Lumbar puncture in children with convulsions associated with fever. *Lancet i*, 785–786.

NATIONAL INSTITUTES OF HEALTH CONSENSUS DEVELOPMENT PANEL (1980) Febrile seizures: long-term management of children with fever-associated seizures. *Br. Med. J.*, **281**, 277–279.

NELSON, K. B., and ELLENBERG, J. H. (1976) Predictors of epilepsy in children who have experienced febrile seizures. *N. Engl. J. Med.*, **295**, 1029–1033.

NELSON, K. B., and ELLENBERG, J. H. (1978) Prognosis in children with febrile seizures. Pediatrics, **61**, 720–727.

PRICHARD, J. S., and MCGREAL, D. A. (1958) Fébrile convulsions. *Med. Clin. North Am.*, **42**, 379–387.

ROLLIN, P., and MASSON, P. (1979) Evaluation de l'investigation des convulsions fébriles. *Union Med. Can.*, **108**, 1–6.

RUTTER, N., and SMALES, O. R. C. (1977) Role of routine investigations in children presenting with their first febrile convulsion. *Arch. Dis. Child.*, **52**, 188–191.

WOLF, S. M. (1978) Laboratory evaluation of the child with a febrile convulsion. *Pediatrics*, **62**, 1074–1076.

Paediatric Perspectives on Epilepsy
Edited by E. Ross and E. Reynolds
© 1985 John Wiley & Sons Ltd.

10

Epilepsy as part of a handicapping condition

JOHN CORBETT
Bethlem Royal Hospital, London

SUMMARY

The relationship between epilepsy and other handicaps can be examined from two different viewpoints. This review first considers the prevalence of epilepsy in various handicapping conditions that involve the central nervous system, mainly above the brainstem. In children with mild mental retardation (IQ 50–70), the prevalence of epilepsy rises from the normal rate (about 0.4%) to 6% for epilepsy of all types. In severe mental retardation (IQ < 50), which is almost invariably associated with brain damage, 30% of affected children have life-long seizures and, in profound retardation (IQ < 20), nearly 50%. Whether or not epilepsy develops seems to depend largely on the nature and site of the cerebral insult and the age at which it occurs.

The second approach is to study the prevalence of handicaps in people with epilepsy, the emphasis here being on behavioural and cognitive impairments. Unexpectedly high rates of intellectual deterioration and behavioural deviance were found recently among children with epilepsy at a special school, despite the use of newer anticonvulsants; the possible reasons for this are discussed.

INTRODUCTION

Epilepsy is, by definition, a symptom of underlying brain dysfunction. Usually there is no gross evidence of structural abnormality detectable on clinical neurological examination. A distinction has sometimes been made between 'organic' and 'complicated' epilepsy, or between 'symptomatic' and 'idiopathic' or 'simple' seizure disorders. Such a classification is helpful in understanding the role of epilepsy as part of a handicapping condition, but it has certain limitations because of our methods of detecting both brain damage and brain dysfunction in clinical situations.

The seizure itself is the most obvious outward manifestation of underlying brain dysfunction and hence structural abnormality. In investigating its nature, no amount of technology can substitute for careful observation, description, and classification of the seizure type and pattern, and of ictal, post-ictal and inter-ictal behavioural events. Such assessment is usually based on the careful interrogation of the patient and witnesses, and it needs to be supplemented in all cases by a painstaking physical examination and psychological assessment. The findings of this diagnostic exercise, applied on an epidemiological scale, provide important evidence concerning the relationships of other handicaps to epilepsy.

PREVALENCE OF EPILEPSY IN HANDICAPPING CONDITIONS

There are two ways of looking at the relationship between epilepsy and other handicaps. The first is to examine the prevalence of epilepsy in various handicapping conditions. The latter can usefully be divided into those with neurological abnormality, distinguishing between lesions above or below the brainstem, and those whose handicapping condition does not involve the nervous system directly. The relationship between various handicaps can then be illustrated by comparison of the association between psychiatric disorders in children whose disability is associated with epilepsy and those in whom it is not (Table I). As one would expect, there is a descending order of frequency, with the highest prevalence of psychiatric disorders being found in patients with brain damage and epilepsy occurring above the brainstem.

Table I   Relationship between handicapping conditions in children and psychiatric disorder (from Rutter et al., 1970)

Handicapping condition	Psychiatric disorder (%)
General population (10–11-year-olds)	6.6
Physical disorders not affecting the nervous system	10.3
Neurological disorders at or below the brainstem	13.3
Uncomplicated epilepsy	28.6
Lesions above the brainstem without fits	37.5
Lesions above the brainstem associated with seizures	58.3

The most obvious handicapping condition associated with brain damage is mental retardation, where the frequency of seizure disorders provides an outward manifestation of the degree of brain involvement (Table II).

The age-specific prevalence rate for established epilepsy in children of school age is approximately 0.4%, if epilepsy is defined as the child having a seizure in the previous year. In children with mild mental retardation, i.e. with an IQ between 50 and 70, the rate rises to 3% for complicated epilepsy and to 6% for epilepsy of all types. The figures for normal and mildly retarded children are from the National Child Development Study (Ross and Peckham, 1983).

Table II   Prevalence of epilepsy in children

National Child Development Study (Ross and Peckham, 1983 Prevalence of epilepsy	0.4%
Febrile convulsions without epileptic sequelae	2.2%
Epilepsy in children with mild mental retardation (IQ 50–70)	6.0%

Epilepsy in children with severe mental retardation (IQ < 50) (Corbett et al., 1975)

	Seizures in past year	Lifelong history of seizures
	19%	32%
IQ 35–50	15%	23%
IQ 20–35	26%	28%
IQ < 20	27%	50%

In severe mental retardation (IQ between 20 and 50), where there is almost invariably an indication of brain damage, the age-specific prevalence rate for epilepsy rises to much higher levels. In our own studies in the Camberwell district of South London, 30% of 145 children who were severely mentally handicapped had a life-long history of seizures, nearly 20% of the cohort under 15 had a history of at least one seizure in the year prior to the study, and 20% were receiving anticonvulsants (Corbett et al., 1975). The frequency of the underlying diagnoses and the seizure rate for each are shown in Table III.

Table III   Percentages of children with seizures for different diagnoses among those with an IQ of less than 50 (from Camberwell Epidemiological Study)

	Number	Seizures (%)
Infections and intoxications	23	34
Trauma and other physical agents	9	33
Metabolic	6	51
Gross brain disease	8	100
Other prenatal causes	16	41
Chromosomal	35	16
Others with family history	13	23
Others with no family history	30	30

In children with profound mental retardation (IQ less than 20), nearly 50% have a life-long history of seizures. We have now followed up the cohort of children who were aged under 14 in 1971 and are now between 14 and 28 years old. As we suspected from the findings of a similar study from Aberdeen (Richardson et al., 1980), we found that epilepsy tends to persist into early adult life, improvements in infantile seizure disorders being balanced by cases of late-onset epilepsy in adolescence.

An adolescent onset of seizures seems particularly likely in children with pervasive developmental disorders who have marked impairments in social relationships, deviant language development (with difficulty in the symbolic and imaginative use of language), and stereotyped, ritualistic behaviour. These are also features of what is known as the autistic syndrome.

It is obviously important to study the occurrence of epilepsy in individual conditions giving rise to mental retardation (Table III). Whether or not epilepsy develops in a particular condition seems to depend largely on the nature and site of the cerebral insult and the age at which it occurs. Epilepsy is, for example, particularly common in the 'phakomatoses'. In tuberous sclerosis and the Sturge–Weber syndrome, epilepsy seems almost inevitable if the subject is severely retarded – and this may well be related to cortical involvement and widespread brain damage. The *type* of epilepsy seems to be largely age dependent, so that tuberous sclerosis frequently presents as infantile spasms, the 'salaam' attacks being a form of myoclonic epilepsy occurring at the stage of development when the child is beginning to sit. Myoclonic astatic attacks are not uncommon if the onset is later, when the child is standing. Both these conditions are usually associated with further intellectual impairment.

It may be that there is no real difference between West's syndrome and the Lennox–Gastaut syndrome, except in the age of onset and the EEG. In West's syndrome the EEG shows the typical picture of hypsarrhythmia, and the somewhat faster high-voltage spike-wave activity is said to be characteristic of the Lennox–Gastaut syndrome. This difference may merely reflect an increase in neurophysiological maturity.

Untreated biochemical abnormalities, such as phenylketonuria, are frequently associated with epilepsy, although this is rare in treated cases. Viral encephalopathies, such as subacute sclerosing panencephalitis and herpes encephalitis, are also frequently associated with characteristic seizure disorders. On the other hand, chromosomal abnormalities such as Down's syndrome, where there is immaturity in brain development but not gross brain damage, are less frequently associated with epilepsy until later life, when Alzheimer-like changes are seen in the brain (Table IV).

The type of secondary handicap associated with retardation has interesting relationships with seizure disorders. Epilepsy is particularly frequent in spastic cerebral palsy (Table V), where seizures occurred in over 60% of subjects studied, and less frequent in perceptual handicaps with deafness and blindness –

Table IV Epilepsy associated with specific mental retardation syndromes

	Epilepsy	West's syndrome	Lennox–Gastaut syndrome
Metabolic abnormalities			
Phenylketonuria	+	+	+
Maple syrup urine disease	+	+	
Hyperornithaemia	+	+	
Isovaleric acidaemia	+	+	
Non-ketotic hyperglycaemia	+	+	
Pyridoxine dependency	+	+	
Leucine-sensitive hypoglycaemia	+	+	+
Tay–Sachs disease	+	+	
Lipoidosis GM_1 and GM_3	+		+
Metachromatic leucodystrophy	+		+
Homocysteinuria			+
Dysplastic conditions			
Tuberous sclerosis	+	+	+
Sturge–Weber syndrome	+	+	+
Megalencephaly	+		+
Other cerebral malformations	+	+	+
Aicardi syndrome	+	+	
Prenatal infections			
Cytomegalovirus	+	+	
Syphilis	+	+	
Toxoplasmosis	+	+	
Postnatal infections			
Purulent meningitis	+		+
Acute encephalitis	+		+
Subacute sclerosing panencephalitis	+		+
Post-immunization encephalopathy	+	+	
Post-traumatic	+		
Chromosomal abnormalities			
Down's syndrome		+	

associated, for example, with rubella embryopathy (Table VI). In mental retardation associated with psychiatric disorders, which tends to be the commonest secondary handicap, seizures are more frequent in hyperkinetic disorders and in the 30% of children who during adolescence are severely retarded with autistic symptoms (Table VII).

It follows from all these considerations that the clinical management of epilepsy in children with mental retardation requires particularly close attention. But, because of our pattern of services, young people with mental retardation

Table V Frequency of major physical and behavioural handicaps, epilepsy and EEG abnormalities

	Cerebral palsy		Severe speech delay		Hyper-kinesis		Psychosis		Stereotypes		Temper		Behaviour disorder	
	No.	%	No.	%	No.	%	No.	%	No.	%	No.	%	No.	%
Epilepsy	30	63	8	17	14	30	7	15	13	27	18	38	19	40
No epilepsy	7	7	32	34	29	31	18	19	35	37	37	39	38	30
EEG abnormal	31	53	12	20	19	32	9	15	21	35	25	42	27	45
EEG normal	1	3	22	57	16	42	19	31	20	52	24	63	22	58
EEG not performed	6	14	8	18	10	23	3	7	6	14	10	23	7	16

Table VI Percentage of children with secondary handicap
who had seizures

	No.	%
No speech	18	33
Severe language disorder	24	17
Severe visual handicap	14	36
Severe deafness	9	22

Table VII Percentage of children with seizures and
psychiatric diagnosis

	No.	%
Childhood psychosis	20	15
Hyperkinetic disorder	18	44
Neurotic disorder	5	20
Conduct disorder	13	30
Severe stereotyped behaviour	7	28
No behaviour disorder	86	30

have frequently been rejected by the paediatric and neurological departments in the past – in favour of children developing more normally. This situation is changing with advances in community care, and epilepsy should no longer be regarded as a reason for hospital inpatient care. But this change does call for major alterations in the pattern of supportive medical services within the community for children with mental handicap. It also represents a revolutionary challenge to paediatric services, where it has so far received little systematic attention. Too many children living at home and in children's homes are still victims of iatrogenic misfortune or therapeutic neglect. A whole range of services is required to support community care, including ready access to outpatient paediatric neurology, anticonvulsant monitoring and a massive education programme for care staff, teachers and parents.

BEHAVIOURAL AND COGNITIVE IMPAIRMENT

An alternative way of looking at epilepsy in relation to other handicaps is to examine the prevalence of such conditions in children with epilepsy. This account will be restricted to behavioural and cognitive impairments, as these are overwhelmingly the most important secondary handicaps.

It has long been recognized that a minority of patients with long-standing epilepsy show progressive intellectual deterioration. The proportion of deteriorated patients does not appear to increase with age, and deteriorated adult patients usually show early indications of this phenomenon in childhood

(Pond, 1961). In some cases of West's syndrome and the Lennox–Gastaut syndrome, status epilepticus and underlying neurodegenerative disorder need to be considered as possible causes, but in other cases there is less evidence of such specific disorders and the aetiology remains obscure.

Early studies suggested that a high seizure frequency was more common in those with intellectual deterioration (Chaudhry and Pond, 1961). However, increasing attention has been paid to the effects of long-term anticonvulsant therapy as a significant and possibly preventable cause of intellectual deterioration (Brown and Reynolds, 1981; Reynolds, 1983).

The general principles of treatment of epilepsy in people with mental retardation are similar to those in non-retarded subjects, but the situation is complicated by several factors. Little is known about the long-term effects of anticonvulsant drugs on the behaviour or intellectual performance of people with mental retardation. The clinical side effects of anticonvulsant medication are often difficult to distinguish from underlying neurological disorders, and seizure disorders are often more complex and severe in the mentally retarded. Evaluation of these effects is further complicated by the polypharmacy often given to severely retarded people with severe and complex epilepsy.

Ideally, research should be prospective, and an increasing number of follow-up studies have been conducted among children with neonatal seizures and those with an onset in the first year of life (Matsumoto *et al.*, 1983; Cavazzuti *et al.*, 1984). New data have also been published on the outlook for infantile spasms (Lombroso, 1983), status epilepticus (Aicardi and Chevrie, 1970), and TLE (Lindsay *et al.*, 1979). These all emphasize the gloomy outlook for such children, but have the disadvantage of referral bias as they are all based on clinic samples.

It is difficult to find epidemiological estimates for the frequency of other handicaps among known epilepsy sufferers. Although one in 10 children may have a seizure at some time during life, the majority are benign and do not lead on to epilepsy. Findings from the British National Development Study suggest that a proportion of the children who had epilepsy needed special schooling and that these had a poor prognosis, but detailed psychological testing was not performed (Ross and Peckham, 1983). The Aarhus studies suggest that only 0.1% suffered from juvenile myoclonic epilepsy; this figure included those with Lennox–Gastaut syndrome (Juul-Jensen and Foldspang, 1983). With older children such studies should ideally be prospective as well as epidemiologically based, and a recent study (Bourgeois *et al.*, 1983) has indeed suggested that 11% of all newly-diagnosed children have a fall of more than 10 points after an average of four years' anticonvulsant therapy. An early age of onset and 'difficult to control' seizures were both found to be predictive of deterioration, and these factors interact.

Retrospective studies are still of value among children showing more severe deterioration, because this is relatively uncommon. We have used a cross-sectional approach to investigate it over an eight-year period in a special school for children with epilepsy. The first study, in 1976, carried out in collaboration with Dr Michael Trimble, showed that 16% of 204 children and adolescents underwent a fall in IQ of more than 15 points (Table VIII) (Corbett and Trimble, 1983). Analysis of the factors which might be incriminated revealed that anticonvulsant therapy, particularly with phenytoin, was most strongly associated with deterioration (probably mediated by folate depletion).

Table VIII   Fall in IQ of children studied in 1976 and 1984 (from Lingfield Hospital School Study)

	1976		1984	
Age range	5–18		5–19	
Mean age	13.2		13.11	
M:F ratio	2.3:1		3:1	
Epilepsy	312		215	
IQ total	311		162	
< 50	67	(21%)	60	(39%)
50–70	121	(38%)	60	(39%)
> 70	123	(39%)	32	(15%)
Sequential IQ scores	204		160	
Fall in IQ > 15 points	32	(16%)	80	(50%)

Preliminary analysis of the data from repeat screening of the population shows that the consumption of phenytoin had declined, and seizure control was better with the newer anticonvulsants (particularly sodium valproate and carbamazepine) and an increased tendency to monotherapy (Table IX). However, the proportion of children with marked intellectual deterioration (by more than 20 points) had increased to 50% of the 160 for whom the results of sequential psychological testing were available. This unexpected finding may be explained in part by selection. Since more children with epilepsy now attend normal schools, the special school takes more severely handicapped children.

Table IX   Anticonvulsants

	1976		1984	
	No.	%	No.	%
Phenobarbitone Primidone	128	(41)	8	(4)
Phenytoin	211	(68)	65	(30)
Sodium valproate	131	(42)	123	(57)
Carbamazepine	132	(42)	110	(51)
Other	173	(57)	88	(41)

It is, however, still important to examine this group of deteriorated children in more detail, and preliminary examination of the data tends to confirm the significance of early seizures, uncontrolled seizures and the mysterious 'Lennox–Gastaut' syndrome as major contributory factors. In addition to the findings on cognitive deterioration, a high rate of behavioural deviance (67%) was noted in this population of children with epilepsy.

Although some relationships were found between individual anticonvulsants and the type of behaviour disorder, and between focal (particularly left temporal) abnormality and individual items of behaviour, there was a striking lack of correlation between the overall deviance scores and other factors such as age at onset of seizures, seizure frequency, IQ, cognitive deterioration, drug administration, blood levels of anticonvulsants and folate levels.

Behavioural deviance might be attributable to interaction between some such factors and psychosocial adversity, which is an important reason for admission to the special school. Unfortunately, information in the latter area was not obtained systematically in 1976, so there are no 'prospective' data on which to base conclusions, but further investigation of the causes of intellectual deterioration and behavioural deviation in this population are currently being undertaken.

REFERENCES

AICARDI, J., and CHEVRIE, J. J. (1970) Convulsive status epilepticus in infants and children. A study of 239 cases. *Epilepsia*, 11, 187–197.
BOURGEOIS, B. F. D., PRENSKY, A. L., PALKES, H. S., TALENT, B. K., and BUSCH, S. G. (1983) Intelligence in epilepsy: A prospective study in children. *Ann. Neurol.*, 14, 438–444.
BROWN, S. W., and REYNOLDS, E. H. (1981) Cognitive impairment in epileptic patients. In: *Epilepsy and Psychiatry*, pp. 147–164 (Eds E. H. Reynolds and M. R. Trimble). Churchill Livingstone, Edinburgh.
CAVAZZUTI, G. B., FERRARI, P., and LALLA, M. (1984) Follow-up study of 482 cases with convulsive disorders in the first year of life. *Dev. Med. Child Neurol.*, 26, 425–437.
CHAUDHRY, M. R., and POND, D. A. (1961) Mental deterioration in epileptic children. *J. Neurol. Neurosurg. Psychiatry*, 24, 213–219.
CORBETT, J. A., HARRIS, R., and ROBINSON, R. (1975) Epilepsy. In: *Mental Retardation and Developmental Disabilities*, VII, pp. 79–111 (Ed. J. Wortis). Bruner Mazel, New York.
CORBETT, J. A., and TRIMBLE, M. R. (1983) Epilepsy and anticonvulsant medication. In: *Developmental Neuropsychiatry*, pp. 112–132 (Ed. M. Rutter). Guildford Press, New York.
JUUL-JENSEN, P., and FOLDSPANG, A. (1983) Natural history of epileptic seizures. *Epilepsia*, 24, 297–312.
LINDSAY, J., OUNSTED, C., and RICHARDS, P. (1979) Long-term outcome in children with temporal lobe seizures. III. Psychiatric aspects in childhood and adult life. *Dev. Med. Child Neurol.*, 21, 631–636.
LOMBROSO, C. T. (1983) A prospective study of infantile spasms: clinical and therapeutic correlations. *Epilepsia*, 24, 135–158.
MATSUMOTO, A., WATANABE, K., SUGIURA, M., NEGORO, T., TAKAESU, E., and IWASE, K. (1983) Long-term prognosis of convulsive disorders in the first year of life: mental and physical development and seizure persistence. *Epilepsia*, 24, 321–329.
POND, D. A. (1961) Psychiatric aspects of epileptic and brain-damaged children. *Br. Med. J.*, 2, 1378–1382.

REYNOLDS, E. H. (1983) Mental effects of antiepileptic medication: A review. *Epilepsia*, **24** (Suppl. 2), 585–595.

RICHARDSON, S. A., KOLLER, H., KATZ, M., and MCLAREN, J. (1980) Seizures and epilepsy in a mentally retarded population over the first 22 years of life. *Appl. Ment. Retard. Res.*, **1**, 123–138.

ROSS, E. M., and PECKHAM, C. S. (1983) School children with epilepsy. In: *Advances in Epileptology. XIVth Epilepsy International Symposium*, pp. 215–220 (Eds M. Parsonage, R. H. E. Grant, A. G. Craig *et al.*). Raven Press, New York.

RUTTER, M., GRAHAM, P., and YULE, W. (1970) A neuropsychiatric study in childhood. *Clinics in Developmental Medicine 35/36*. Heinemann, London.

Paediatric Perspectives on Epilepsy
Edited by E. Ross and E. Reynolds
© 1985 John Wiley & Sons Ltd.

11

Selection of school for children with epilepsy

LEON POLNAY
Queen's Medical Centre, University of Nottingham

SUMMARY

Most children with epilepsy can attend ordinary schools, but some require special education. This calls for formal assessment and a statement of special educational needs. Under the procedures laid down by the Department of Education and Science in 1983, parental involvement is followed by educational, medical and psychological advice, to determine the relevant aspects of the child's functioning, the aims to which provision should be directed, and the facilities required to promote the achievement of these objectives. The statement is reviewed annually and the child reassessed in the early teens. Effective communication is necessary between school doctors, nurses, teachers and parents, bearing in mind that factors other than fits determine the need for special education.

The choice of school is an important decision for every parent. For the majority of children, this process is completed quite satisfactorily without professional interference. For a minority, formal assessment procedures are followed. Designated under the 1981 Education Act as requiring 'provision additional to, or otherwise different from the resources generally available in ordinary schools in the area under normal arrangements', these result in the issue of a 'statement of special education needs'. In jargon, the child is 'statemented', in contrast to being 'ascertained' under the previous regulations. I suspect that, for many, not too much has changed in terms of final placements, but that the method of reaching decisions has become somewhat more lengthy and complicated. The chief principles of the procedure (Department of Education and Science, 1983) are as follows:

1. Parental involvement
2. Seeking educational, medical and psychological advice, aimed at
    determining:
    (i)   the relevant aspects of the child's functioning, including his strengths
          and weaknesses, his relation with his environment at home and at
          school, and any relevant aspects of his past history
    (ii) the aims to which provision for the child should be directed to enable
          him to develop educationally and increase his independence
    (iii) the facilities and resources recommended to promote the achievement
          of these aims
3. Placement in an ordinary school, provided this is compatible with:
    (i)   his receiving the special educational facilities that he requires
    (ii) the provision of efficient education for the children with whom he
          will be taught
    (iii) the efficient use of resources
4. Annual review of the statement
5. Reassessment between the ages of 13½ and 14½.

It is fortunate that the majority of children with epilepsy fall outside these
procedures. However, for every child, there needs to be effective communication

Table I Numbers of handicapped pupils, by category and placement (England and
Wales, 1979)

Category	Attending special schools	Awaiting admission to special schools	In special classes in ordinary schools	In other places*	Total
Blind	1 021	31	8	20	1 080
Partially sighted	2 152	72	154	11	2 389
Deaf	3 529	52	292	32	3 905
Partially hearing	2 092	143	3 474	70	5 779
Speech defect	1 134	161	799	156	2 250
Autistic	796	30	89	62	977
Educationally subnormal					
Mild	62 495	3530	8 330	271	74 626
Severe	30 643	685	212	638	32 178
Physically handicapped	13 654	386	473	727	15 240
Delicate	5 199	271	321	384	6 175
Epileptic	981	24	80	24	1 109
Maladjusted	15 752	1522	1 548	2458	21 280
All categories	139 448	6907	15 780	4853	166 988

*Hospitals, other units (e.g. units for spastics) and home.

between school doctors, nurses, teachers and parents. Much of educational medicine is really 'liaison paediatrics'.

The National Child Development Study (Ross *et al.*, 1980) gave prevalence figures of 4.5 per 1000 of active epilepsy and of 0.5 per 1000 of serious epileptic problems in the 11-year-olds whom they studied. Based on a school and pre-school population of 18 000 000, about 9000 children will have serious epileptic problems. However, under the previous categories of special education, only 1109 children were included in 1979, but it seems likely that others will have been placed under other headings (Table I). In the NCDS figures, 43 of the 64 children with epilepsy were attending ordinary schools and 21 received special educational provision. At 16 years, 22 were receiving special education, of whom 11 were ESN (moderate), four were ESN (severe), two were at school for physical handicap, four were in special residential schools for epilepsy, and one was at home (Ross *et al.*, 1983).

It is clear from this and other studies (e.g. Kurtz, 1982) that factors other than the presence of fits are responsible for the need for special education. These may be physical or mental handicap, sensory handicap, behavioural problems (Stores, 1978) or social problems. Not all children with the same handicap are equal. The parents' ability to cope and their need for support may overshadow the child's needs and the school's ability to educate him.

Although, at 11 years old, the children in the NCDS with epilepsy had poorer scores in reading and mathematics than controls, and were more likely to have prolonged absences from school, at 16 years there was no significant difference in attainment for those at ordinary schools.

WHAT ARE THE NEEDS OF THE CHILD AND HIS FAMILY?

The first need is for comprehensive assessment. In view of the wide range of learning, behavioural and other problems described above, control of the fits represents only a small part of the management. In addition to the paediatrician, this might involve the educational psychologist, social worker, speech therapist and other medical and paramedical colleagues. It is essential to have effective communication and integration of the medical, social and educational input (Polnay and Hull, 1985).

Secondly, continuity of care is important from all those in contact with the family. This is sometimes the exception rather than the rule and, as the notes grow, individual knowledge about the child and family may actually decrease. They may then meet a series of strangers who are expected to advise one another constructively about the needs of the child. If counselling is to be effective, a trusting relationship must first be allowed to develop.

Thirdly, there must be access to care. The family and the child must be able to get help rapidly when they need it, for example if there is an increase in fit frequency.

WHAT ARE THE NEEDS OF THE SCHOOL?

Teachers in general will not have received any instruction on childhood illnesses during their training. Yet they will meet many health problems in their classes. With the move to integrate more handicapped children into ordinary schools, the need for information on child health issues will increase. Teachers might feel that it is wise to hold pressure off the child with epilepsy, to apply different levels of discipline or have lower expectations of achievement than for other children (Bower, 1978). But this could lead to poor attainments which would not help in the unequal struggle for employment at school leaving.

The following is offered to teachers as a framework of medical advice on a child with epilepsy:
1. Name the condition.
2. Describe what this means *in lay terms*.
3. Provide a problem list of the identified difficulties that the child has.
4. List and explain any treatment that the child is receiving, particularly anything that is required to be done in school. In the case of medication, teachers need precise information on dose and warning of any side effects that might occur. In this way problems may be reported early and undesirable action, e.g. punishment of the child, avoided. Teachers need not only to be informed initially of the child's treatment but also kept up to date with any major changes that take place.
5. The teacher needs to be informed of what to do if the child has a fit in the classroom, in order to avoid overzealous first aid, panic, or the child being frequently sent home or parents summoned.
6. The teachers need advice on what restrictions, if any, are necessary. Without guidance, the school might opt for safety and unnecessarily restrict what the child is allowed to do. The advice must of course relate to the individual; a list to cover all children with epilepsy is highly undesirable. However, in general, children should be allowed to swim with supervision – the risks are very low. Restriction of off-the-floor gym exercises is relevant for some children, but ordinary team sports are acceptable (O'Donohoe, 1983).
7. Before leaving school, advice will be needed on choice of career. Counselling of the child and family, and liaison with career officers might be necessary.

REFERENCES

Bower, B. (1978) The treatment of epilepsy in children. *Br. J. Hosp. Med.,* **19,** 8–23.
Department of Education and Science (1983) Assessment and statement of special educational needs. Circular 1/83.
Kurtz, Z. (1982) Special schooling for children with epilepsy. In: *Research Progress in Epilepsy,* pp. 538–546 (Ed. F. C. Rose). Pitman Medical, London.
O'Donohoe, N. V. (1983) What shall the child with epilepsy be allowed to do? *Arch. Dis. Child.,* **58,** 934–937.

POLNAY, L., and HULL, D. (1985) Chapters on longstanding illness and educational medicine. In: *Community Paediatrics*, in press. Churchill Livingstone, Edinburgh.

ROSS, E. M., PECKHAM, C. S., WEST, P. B., and BUTLER, N. R. (1980) Epilepsy in childhood: findings from the National Child Development Study. *Br. Med. J.*, 1, 207–210.

ROSS, E. M., KURTZ, Z., and PECKHAM, C. S. (1983) Children with epilepsy: Implications for the school health service. *Public Health*, **93**, 75–81.

STORES, G. (1978) School children with epilepsy at risk for learning and behavioural problems. *Dev. Med. Child Neurol.*, **20**, 502–508.

Discussion

Dr A. J. Franklin (Chelmsford): In relation to the intellectual deterioration you noted in children on anticonvulsants, Dr Corbett, some years ago it was suggested that vitamin B can help to reverse this. Have you any comments?

Corbett: Vitamin B_6 (pyridoxine) is an interesting substance in disabling myoclonic epilepsy, as noted in my paper. In certain situations, for example Down's syndrome with myoclonic epilepsy of late onset, it does seem to be helpful, and possibly in Down's children with infantile spasms. But we have not considered vitamin B in mental deterioration, which is notoriously hard to assess. Records are often poor, and it may be impossible to find out, for example, how long the developing brain was subjected to phenytoin or phenobarbitone, what the seizure frequency was, why drug changes were made, and so on. In a cohort of 80 children we are starting to study, research is going to be extremely difficult. We are planning to look at growth, because they seem to be small, to interview the families in detail, where I suspect we may get better records than from hospital notes, and to investigate them both neurophysiologically and in some cases with NMR scanning. We wonder if repeated head blows from myoclonic astatic epilepsy may have caused some of the deterioration, perhaps because of inadequate head protection. Among other factors, arylsulphatase deficiency may play a part in some of these children, and we would be very grateful for any suggestions.

Dr S. H. Green (Birmingham): All of us come across syndromes which are difficult to classify, children whom we believe have epilepsy but whose EEG is either mildly abnormal or completely normal. I would like to ask Professor Aicardi how much he relies on the EEG in diagnosing such syndromes.

Aicardi: Basically the diagnosis has to be clinical but there is no question that the EEG, when it is positive – which is not always the case – does add something to the clinical diagnosis. Certainly the delineation of epileptic syndromes in childhood has to be partly clinical and partly electroencephalographic. I should emphasize that a number of epilepsies in childhood, especially in younger infants and children, are extremely difficult or impossible to classify, including many cases with partial epilepsies in early childhood and infancy and the majority of cases of grand mal epilepsies, which do not really belong to any syndrome. But of course there are children with the most dreadful epilepsies who have perfectly normal EEGs for years and years. They are also quite difficult to treat.

Dr T. H. J. Matthews (Romford): May I ask Dr Addy how long children with a febrile convulsion should remain in hospital – until the fever has abated or 24 hours later?

Addy: Should the child be in hospital in the first place? That depends on the qualities of the general practitioner, the social circumstances, and the readiness of the parents to look after the child and report to the general practitioner if things are not right. Admission is not necessary in all circumstances. Where I work, in an inner city, most children are brought up to the casualty department, bypassing the general practitioner anyway. My own practice is to keep children in hospital at least 24 hours, because if they are going to have another convulsion they will probably have it within that time. After 24 hours, if the temperature is settling, not necessarily down to normal, the child is well, and we are convinced he does not have meningitis, then I allow him home.

Dr G. P. McMullin (Warrington): Professor Aicardi's delineation of the five ages of epilepsies is extremely useful, but I really wonder whether the statement that children with seizures in the first year of life have a poor prognosis is always justified. I am thinking particularly of the paper by O'Brien *et al.* (1981) which showed that most children having seizures in the first year of life after the neonatal period have a good prognosis. This would be my experience, also working in a district general hospital. What Douglas Addy said about selection and published studies emanating from centres of excellence, where only the more difficult cases are seen, is probably biasing the specialist attitude to seizures at this age.

Aicardi: I certainly agree that the factor of selection is a very important one. Concerning epilepsies in the first year, a recent paper by Ellenberg *et al.* (1984) about children with epilepsy during the first year of life showed that the prognosis is not nearly as bad as we have usually thought. Nonetheless, even in this paper, which concludes that there is no difference between first-year epilepsy and later epilepsy (which I cannot really accept), a close look at the figures will reveal that there is indeed a difference, though less marked than the one we see in selected samples. I still believe that having epilepsy before the age of one year is more dangerous than might be expected from our own figures, which are undoubtedly biased.

Dr B. D. Bower (Oxford): Don't you think that one of the factors that comes into this question is the difficulty in distinguishing between fits, faints and funny turns in the first six months?

Aicardi: There is also a tendency for pathology to evolve with the times. In a country like France 15 years ago there were a number of cases of long-lasting febrile convulsions leaving sequelae. Now we don't see them any longer. Two recent MD theses on this topic, in Marseilles and Lyons, both show a dramatic decrease of long-lasting febrile convulsions with sequelae over the past 15 years. This may not be true of other countries or other periods.

Addy: I am not entirely convinced that rectal diazepam is useful, but pharmacologically there is reason to believe that it works.

O'Donohoe: Dr Corbett raised the question of protective helmets. What we need in my experience is a helmet that protects the face, chin and teeth as well as the head.

Corbett: The main need is surely to protect the cranium. A type of foam originally devised by NASA for the nose cones of space rockets is now being used by Remploy in their vitrithene helmets. This material has a remarkably high degree of impact absorbancy. Quite a thin layer, about 5 mm thick, lining a helmet will protect the cranium. With a bit of thought helmets can be made to look much more cosmetic than they do. But the main point is that we do not know the effect of these repeated blows, particularly the contrecoup injury from repeated blows on the back of the head from falling backwards. In front, the nose protects the brain to some extent, but I wonder how important falling backwards repeatedly may be in causing subsequent intellectual impairment – the 'punch-drunk' syndrome.

Aicardi: I do not really know, but it might well be important. Clearly when these children fall 50 times a day, and sometimes get severe injuries and coma when they fall, the effect could be serious.

Corbett: That is one of the things we hope to settle by imaging studies.

REFERENCES

ELLENBERG, J. H., HIRTZ, D. G., and NELSON, K. B. (1984) Age of onset of seizures in young children. *Ann. Neurol.*, **15**, 127–134.

O'BRIEN, T., COUNAHAN, R., O'BRIEN, B., and COSGROVE, J. F. (1981) Prognosis of convulsions between one and six months of age. *Arch. Dis. Child.*, **56**, 643–644.

Part IV: The schoolchild

Paediatric Perspectives on Epilepsy
Edited by E. Ross and E. Reynolds
© 1985 John Wiley & Sons Ltd.

12

Types of epilepsy in the young schoolchild: stress, flicker and nocturnal seizures

ORVAR EEG-OLOFSSON
Department of Paediatrics, University Hospital, Linköping, Sweden

SUMMARY

Many children have seizures which mimic epilepsy but cannot be classified as such; examples include tics, headache, abdominal pain, vomiting, sleep disturbances, aggressive outbursts and hysterical reactions. EEG manifestations suggestive of epilepsy are also found in normal children. Among nearly 750 children studied, 2.4% had spike and wave activity during wakefulness and light sleep, 9% had generalized spike and wave complexes and bitemporo-occipital paroxysmal responses to intermittent photic stimulation, and 8% had diffuse bilateral synchronous paroxysmal activity during drowsiness and light sleep. Such clinical and EEG findings need to be carefully distinguished from findings in true epilepsy. *Stress, flicker* and *sleep* may act as provoking mechanisms in young schoolchildren susceptible to seizures, producing various types of seizure. Nocturnal epilepsy, for example, may take the form of *atonic myoclonic* fits, *'absences'*, sometimes associated with myoclonic jerks of the face, shoulders and arms, or *benign epilepsy of childhood with centro-temporal EEG foci*, which accounts for about 15% of all epilepsy in childhood. Carbamazepine (Tegretol®) is the treatment of choice for this last form, which has a very good prognosis.

INTRODUCTION

Between the ages of five and 11 years, the young schoolchild is in a period of life usually characterized as comparatively harmonious. Towards the end of it, the child has normally achieved an optimum of adaption, his maturation and behaviour naturally being influenced by genetic mechanisms and

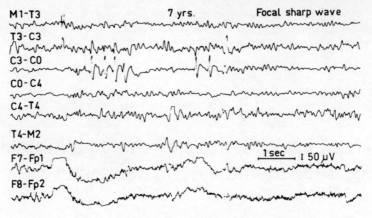

Fig. 1 Focal sharp waves recorded at rest

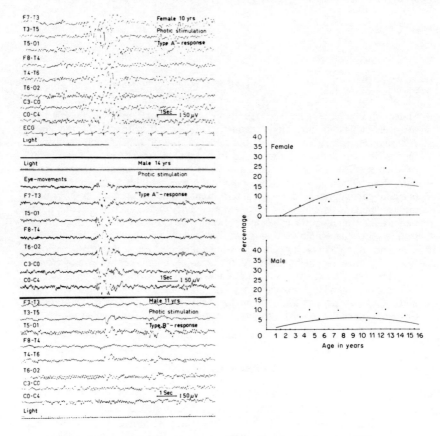

Fig. 2 Paroxysmal responses to intermittent photic stimulation

environmental factors. The prevalence of epilepsy in this age group is approximately 0.6%.

This paper concentrates on epilepsy appearing in response to stress, to flickering or sudden flashing of light and during sleep in the young mentally normal schoolchild. First, it is important to note that children quite frequently have disorders which simulate epilepsy but cannot be classified as such. Examples are syncope, tics, headache, abdominal pain, vomiting, sleep disturbances, outbursts of aggressiveness, and hysterical reactions. These individuals may show paroxysmal electroencephalographic manifestations, which can also be found in completely normal children. The occurrence of paroxysmal activity in the EEG of 743 selected healthy and normal children has been described by Eeg-Olofsson et al. (1971). Focal spikes and sharp waves and focal spike-like activity during wakefulness and sleep was found in 2.4%, mainly young schoolchildren (Fig. 1). During intermittent photic stimulation, bilateral synchronous generalized spike and wave complexes and bitemporo-occipital paroxysmal responses were found in 9.0% overall, but significantly more in girls than boys, and among the girls significantly more during and after puberty than before (Fig. 2). Finally, during drowsiness and light sleep, diffuse bilateral synchronous

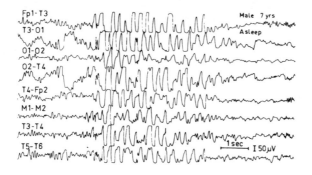

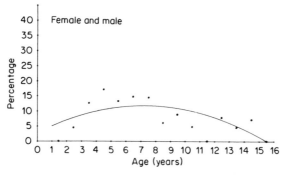

Fig. 3 Diffuse, bilateral synchronous paroxysmal activity during light sleep

paroxysmal activity, in the form of slow waves intermingled with small spikes, was found in 8.0%, mainly young schoolchildren (Fig. 3). It is important that clinical symptoms are carefully evaluated in relation to age, psychosocial factors etc., and that the findings are weighed against the abnormal EEG, which must be judged in relation to age, alertness and background activity.

STRESS SEIZURES

Seizures during stress are not very common in this age group, and significantly less common during childhood as a whole compared with adults. Now and then, however, precipitating factors such as physical and mental overstrain, intense fear, pain or rage may trigger seizures in a predisposed child with any kind of epilepsy. Worry and anxiety over problems at school and at home, such as the prospect of a move to a new school or a new class, or parental illness often act in the same way. Minor medical manipulations, like blood tests, dental treatment or minor surgical operations, may also trigger a seizure. But when a child is faced with a single stress factor with which he is competent to deal he does not get a fit. It is also rare for children to have fits during examinations. A child is liable to have a seizure, however, when exposed to an environment with which he cannot cope. To avoid the risk of stress seizures the following rules may be of importance: obtain careful information about seizures, medication, side effects of drugs, etc.; in connection with the onset of epilepsy, give monotherapy if possible; and avoid drugs giving rise to behaviour disturbances.

FLICKER SEIZURES

Flicker or photic-induced seizures are attacks provoked by flickering or sudden flashing of light. They may occur in children with different types of epilepsy or may be the only manifestation of a seizure disorder (for review, see Newmark and Penry, 1979). Flicker seizures are usually associated with a photoconvulsive response in the EEG (Fig. 4). This response may show generalized irregular 2.5–3.5 Hz spike and wave activity, or generalized polyspikes, or polyspikes and waves. Abnormal photic responses occur in patients with a variety of seizure disorders.

Photosensitivity is age and sex dependent and also related to genetic factors. The median age for the occurrence of photic-induced seizures is 11–15 years, with a predominance of girls. According to Jeavons and Harding (1975) the ratio of girls to boys is about 3:2. With respect to genetic factors, photosensitivity has often been observed in more than one family member. Although a photoconvulsive response in the EEG is common in family members, particularly in the younger ones, photic-induced epilepsy is much less prevalent. Its presence in several families studied does however suggest a genetic trait. Twin studies

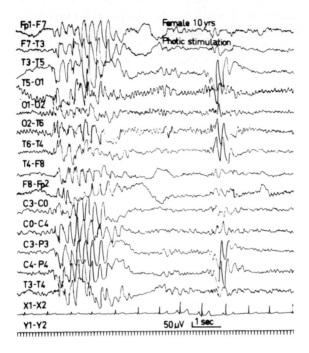

Fig. 4 Photoconvulsive response

strengthen the evidence for a genetic trait, as the concordance for seizures is 100% (Jeavons and Harding, 1975). Several reports confirm that photoconvulsive responses and photic-induced seizures have occurred throughout many generations of the same family. The inheritance pattern is not consistent but, as in other types of epilepsy, a polygenic mechanism is most probable. The prognosis of photosensitive epileptic children is good and is said not to affect the prognosis for future seizures at all. Recovery is unlikely before the age of 18 years.

Television-induced seizures

Television is the commonest precipitant of seizures, giving rise to a pleasurable sensation in some children. Usually the type of fit provoked by TV-light is a tonic-clonic seizure, sometimes preceded by myoclonic jerking. Repetitive flickering at discotheques, now and then patronized by the oldest children in this age group, and home movies are also possible trigger mechanisms for photic-induced seizures.

Self-induced seizures

Other methods of producing seizures are hand-waving and repeated blinking in front of a light source. However, it is important to differentiate between provoking mechanisms and seizure equivalents. For example, a child thought to be self-inducing seizures actually had seizures consisting of hand movements and alternating deviations of the eyes and head. Self-induced seizures usually occur at somewhat younger ages than other photosensitivity; they are also more prevalent in children with slight mental retardation.

Therapy

A careful history, knowledge of the personality of the child and general information is important. To watch TV, the child should sit about three metres from the set at an angle of 45°. It is important to have light in the room and behind the TV set. Ordinary or possibly polarized sunglasses are recommended for outdoor use in sunny weather. Most photosensitive children do not need anticonvulsant therapy, but those with spike and wave discharges in their resting EEG should be treated. Sodium valproate is the drug of choice.

NOCTURNAL SEIZURES

Many nocturnal seizures undoubtedly go unrecognized or unreported. When parents go to see a doctor after their child has suffered a nocturnal fit, it will probably not be the very first one. Nocturnal seizures tend to occur either within the first few hours after going to sleep, mainly during deep sleep, or one to two hours before the usual awakening time, mainly during lighter sleep. Seizures occuring a few minutes to about one hour after awakening, so-called early morning seizures, can be included in this category. It is also important to consider non-epileptic disorders, which can simulate epilepsy, for instance disorders of arousal, such as nocturnal enuresis, sleep talking, sleep walking (somnambulism), night terrors (pavor nocturnus), and sleep jerks. Disorders of real sleep, particularly involving dream or REM sleep, are narcolepsy and nightmares.

It is also important to recognize the different paroxysmal EEG phenomena that normally occur during drowsiness and the different stages of sleep. Such phenomena are for instance vertex sharp waves, humps and K-complexes. Certain clinical manifestations and EEG patterns of this kind can mislead the doctor, causing him to prescribe unnecessary anticonvulsant therapy.

Diagnostic features of nocturnal seizures include, for example, a witnessed focal or generalized tonic or clonic attack, waking with a bitten tongue, waking with a disordered bed, and post-ictal phenomena such as headache or Todd's paresis.

Atonic-myoclonic epilepsy

This is often associated with nocturnal fits, especially during the deeper stages of sleep. Drop attacks usually appear as early morning seizures.

Absence epilepsy

Seizures connected with absence epilepsy, also called primary generalized corticoreticular epilepsy, occur mainly in the daytime, but absences and especially myoclonic jerks of the face, shoulders and arms are sometimes seen as early morning seizures.

Benign epilepsy of children with centro-temporal EEG foci

This is the most common type of epilepsy manifesting itself in sleep (Blom *et al.*, 1972). It was first described by Nayrac and Beaussart (1958) and represents about 15% of all types of epilepsy in childhood. The seizures are partial with a strong tendency to generalization. Other descriptive names for the same types of fit are 'Sylvian seizures and midtemporal spike foci' (Lombroso, 1967) and 'chuckling and glugging seizures at night' (Bladin and Papworth, 1974). An autosomal dominant gene with age-dependent penetrance is believed to be responsible for the EEG trait, which is very characteristic (the same as Fig. 1). This benign type of epilepsy mainly appears between five and 11 years of age.

Even if the EEG pattern is inherited as an autosomal dominant trait, the clinical manifestations do not appear to follow the same rule. As in the case of epilepsy with absences or photic-induced seizures, this type of epilepsy is polygenically determined and thus has a multifactorial background. One of these factors may be a defective immune mechanism. Eeg-Olofsson *et al.* (1982) showed that children with this type of seizure and their parents had a statistically significant low incidence of the HLA A1, B8 haplotype compared to controls. This haplotype is the most common one in all populations and thus probably offers some kind of biological advantage, perhaps as a carrier of protector genes against certain noxious agents, such as infectious organisms. Lack of this haplotype could therefore explain a lowered immunological defensive mechanism, resulting in increased risk for the appearance of a seizure disorder. The mechanism is probably genetically determined.

For treatment of 'benign epilepsy of children with centro-temporal EEG foci' the drug of choice is carbamazepine (Tegretol®), and the prognosis is very good (Blom and Heijbel, 1982).

CONCLUSION

Epilepsy in childhood, between the ages of five and 11 years, can manifest itself in response to provoking mechanisms, notably stress, flicker and especially sleep. It is important for the doctor to know of the differential diagnoses, especially those concerning behavioural disorders, and also to be able to recognize EEG patterns of epileptogenic or other paroxysmal kind, which can also appear in normal children.

REFERENCES

BLADIN, P. F., and PAPWORTH, G. (1974) Chuckling and glugging seizures at night – Sylvian spike epilepsy. *Proc. Aust. Assoc. Neurol.,* **11**, 171–176.

BLOM, S., and HEIJBEL, J. (1982) Benign epilepsy of children with centro-temporal EEG foci: A follow-up study in adulthood of patients initially studied as children. *Epilepsia,* **23**, 629–632.

BLOM, S., HEIJBEL, J., and BERGFORS, P. G. (1972) Benign epilepsy of children with centro-temporal EEG foci. *Epilepsia,* **13**, 609–619.

EEG-OLOFSSON, O., PETERSEN, I., and SELLDEN, U. (1971) The development of the electroencephalogram in normal children from the age of 1 through 15 years. Paroxysmal activity. *Neuropaediatrie,* **2**, 375–404.

EEG-OLOFSSON, O., SÄFWENBERG, J., and WIGERTZ, A. (1982) HLA and epilepsy: An investigation of different types of epilepsy in children and their families. *Epilepsia,* **23**, 27–34.

JEAVONS, P. M., and HARDING, F. A. (1975) *Photosensitive Epilepsy. A Review of the Literature and a Study of 460 Patients.* Heinemann, London.

LOMBROSO, C. T. (1967) Sylvian seizures and midtemporal spike foci in children. *Arch. Neurol.,* **17**, 52–59.

NAYRAC, P., and BEAUSSART, M. (1958) Les pointes-ondes prérolandiques: Expression EEG très particulière. Etude électroclinique de 21 cas. *Rev. Neurol.,* **99**, 201–206.

NEWMARK, M. E., and PENRY, J. K. (1979) *Photosensitivity and Epilepsy: A Review.* Raven Press, New York.

Paediatric Perspectives on Epilepsy
Edited by E. Ross and E. Reynolds
© 1985 John Wiley & Sons Ltd.

13

Hospital investigation of a child with epilepsy

IAN McKINLAY
Booth Hall Children's Hospital, Manchester

SUMMARY

When childhood epilepsy has been diagnosed clinically it should be investigated fully, but in doubtful cases the indications for investigation are less clear. The high cost may be disproportionate to the benefit, and anxiety may be created unnecessarily. Single seizures or febrile convulsions may not require further investigations if the child is normal on clinical examination. If CNS infection is suspected, lumbar puncture should be considered. An EEG is indicated after recurrent seizures, as it may assist localization and classification of the seizure type. Skull X-rays are seldom positive. If the timing of seizures suggests hypoglycaemia, the blood sugar should be determined. CAT scanning and other special investigations are required only in selected cases. Control of anticonvulsant drug therapy can be greatly assisted by determination of serum or saliva concentrations. All investigations should be done for good reasons – and explained, so far as possible, to children with epilepsy and their parents.

INTRODUCTION

Children are commonly investigated for *possible* epilepsy, perhaps partly because doctors themselves fear it. But what impact does the process of investigation have on the child and family when the suspected diagnosis is not confirmed? Such children disappear from our follow-up – we are 'glad to say that our tests have excluded epilepsy'. But who asked us to include it? And are the patients grateful that we did so? If they were worried by a family history of fits, some may of course be glad that the tests were carried out. The child's view of the investigative process is largely unknown, and unsolicited. For vulnerable children in difficult predicaments, investigation can promote an interest in illness as a 'career'. Infants and children who are not aware of the behaviour they are reported to demonstrate, such as brief absences, may be mystified by the exercise. They may be frightened by it too. Consequences of adverse reaction to 'negative investigations' may not become evident to the hospital physician who ordered them – but trouble the family, the child guidance services, the general practitioner or the child psychiatrist.

A neurology department like ours sees selected children, often referred by other consultants, with a 'diagnosis' of epilepsy. A quarter of such referred children are not considered to have epilepsy when seen in the outpatient department, and are not investigated for the condition – although this opinion can turn out to be incorrect occasionally. The decision to investigate epilepsy is a responsibility that should be entertained only when there are clear clinical indications that a child has had recurrent epileptic seizures. In other words, the clinical diagnosis should first be established.

Of all children admitted to our ward, three out of every seven are for investigation of epilepsy. Their mean length of stay is four days, compared with a regional mean of five days. However, a small core – about 10% – occupy nearly half our patient-bed days. Most of these are infants with refractory seizures. They represent some of the most challenging problems of paediatric care, usually with such disappointing prognosis as to justify major reappraisal of our knowledge of causes and treatments. Perhaps the lack of interest in such children has stemmed from the fact that most of them develop severe mental handicap – yet this could be an even stronger argument for further research (Chevrie and Aicardi, 1978).

The cost of investigation has not been a major issue in the National Health Service, because it has not been known and no charges are made. Development of clinical budgeting may change this in our current climate of cash limits and recession, with the emphasis on district rather than regional services. Hospital doctors are being forced to consider 'value for money' because resources to employ staff, to pay for tests and to buy equipment are all limited.

In the neurology department of our children's hospital, the average four-day admission of a child with possible epilepsy currently costs £350. For infants with proven complex seizure disorders the average admission lasts 30 days and costs £2500. Cost-benefit analysis has not been carried out but we must accept that some of these patients leave hospital in a similar state to that in which they entered. If costs of depreciation and maintenance of equipment are included in estimating the expense of investigation, as well as staff salaries and consumables, the amounts are found to range from nearly £20 for a standard EEG (which, in our department, routinely includes hyperventilation and photic stimulation) to nearly £70 for a peripatetic recording (Table I).

Those of us involved in organizing neurophysiology departments for children need to be aware of such costs in negotiating with our health authorities, who

Table I   EEG costs for children

Type of EEG	Total cost per test	Depreciation and maintenance per test
Standard	£18.29	£ 2.13
Sleep	£56.42	£ 7.77
Peripatetic	£68.18	£31.01
Portable	£49.92	£ 7.77
Ocular compression	£33.25	£ 2.13

still lack mechanisms to allow for depreciation and maintenance costs. When equipment needs to be replaced it often provokes a funding crisis at present, but this need not be so.

Important though these housekeeping isssues are, they should not deflect us from understanding that appropriate investigation, accurate diagnosis and good communication with parents and children can lead to considerable relief from sickness, improvement in life prospects, and thus substantial financial savings, when compared with the effects of neglect or errors.

INVESTIGATIVE PROCEDURE

The doctor examining a child reported to have had 'fits' needs to take account of the differential diagnosis (British Medical Journal, 1979), including forms of syncope, paroxysmal vertigo, tantrums, night terrors, breath-holding and psychogenic phenomena. Obtaining a thorough clinical description of the circumstances and nature of the episodes is itself a fundamental part of the investigation. A family history is vital, not only in reaching a provisional diagnosis but in understanding the significance of the episodes for the family. Auntie may be said to have 'died in a fit', or perhaps a cousin with fits is known to be mentally handicapped.

The child who has had a single seizure should be examined for general physical abnormalities, such as depigmented or pigmented skin lesions, and neurodevelopmental problems. Whereas one child in 200 in the general population experiences epilepsies (Baumann *et al.*, 1978), one in three mentally handicapped or cerebral-palsied children is affected and may present with a fit. If the examination is satisfactory we often feel that no further investigation is necessary, even if the single seizure has been prolonged (not 'status' but lasting more than 10 minutes) or focal. If seizures have been provoked by fever, investigations are very unlikely to be helpful, except when the child's clinical state suggests infection of the nervous system; lumbar puncture is then indicated. In selected children CAT scanning should be considered, for example if encephalitis or cerebral abscess is suspected. In such children a scan should precede lumbar puncture.

If the child has had recurrent seizures, thought to be of cerebral origin, EEG is useful for localization and classification of seizure type. Skull X-ray offers such a low yield of positive results that it is not our usual practice to request one. When the seizures have occurred before breakfast, after prolonged fasting or, in infants, soon after a milk feed, investigation for hypoglycaemia is appropriate, but not as a routine. In general, estimation of serum calcium and electrolytes is unproductive. If seizures are frequent, however, these will be requested, together with amino acid chromatography and porphyrin assay in urine. Virological investigation will identify occasional infants who have suffered intrauterine infection.

ELECTROENCEPHALOGRAPHY

Although epilepsy is traditionally a clinical diagnosis, it is wise to beware of making it in a child whose EEG is persistently normal, especially if a tracing soon after an episode does not show post-ictal features. Peripatetic EEG investigation has undoubtedly helped to clarify this, however. For a child whose resting EEG is unhelpful but who experiences frequent attacks of an uncertain nature this technique can record the EEG activity at the time of the episodes (Stores, 1984). Conversely, the majority of children who show focal 'epileptic' EEG discharges do not suffer from epilepsy (Eeg-Olofsson et al., 1971; Bernardina and Beghini, 1976; Lerman and Kivity-Ephraim, 1981). Some EEG appearances do correlate well with a clinical diagnosis (e.g. hypsarrhythmia in infantile spasms, or periodic paroxysmal high-voltage slow-wave activity in subacute sclerosing panencephalitis), but clinical features should always be considered together with EEG findings (Beaussart, 1972).

EEG tracings taken during sleep can be informative in highlighting focal abnormalities and in clarifying seizure type, for example in benign rolandic epilepsy or Lennox-Gastaut syndrome. They may show 'electrical status' during sleep in some psychotic children. One method used for inducing sleep is prior sleep deprivation, which is attractive because it is physiological but there can be practical difficulties. Other departments use drugs such a chlorpromazine or sodium amytal. The former is theoretically risky because it is convulsant and it could be argued that abnormalities activated by it are difficult to interpret. By contrast, a barbiturate, being anticonvulsant, could be thought to suppress seizure activity. In practice I know of no serious difficulties from using such drugs, but it would be interesting to compare the results obtained after different methods of obtaining a sleep recording. I have seen children who had fits following trimeprazine sedation and would not recommend using it for sleep records.

An EEG has some predictive value when obtained at the time drug withdrawal is being considered. However, as an abnormal tracing would not dissuade me from offering to withdraw treatment I do not obtain one routinely.

Certain clinical problems present investigative difficulties. The young child with frequent fits, especially myoclonus, may have a degenerative disorder of the CNS or 'only' refractory epilepsy. To clarify the aetiological diagnosis, assay of lysosomal enzymes or tissue biopsies may need to be considered. In most cases there is time to allow the clinical features to clarify themselves, but when genetic counselling is required, earlier investigation may be justified.

COMPUTER-ASSISTED TOMOGRAPHY

CAT scanning is not usually indicated for children with epilepsies, but the positive yield in certain groups justifies the investigation. Children with infantile spasms commonly show abnormalities, such as atrophy or periventricular calcification, before treatment is initiated (Singer et al., 1982). The calcified lesions in those with tuberous sclerosis may not appear until the second year of life, however, so that both an initial and a follow-up scan may be indicated. In children with persistently focal fits and focal neurological signs (e.g. cerebral palsy), the scan yield is quite high but the treatment implications are slight. When a scan is obtained its main value is to facilitate exploration. If surgery is being considered for a child with focal fits but not neurological signs, a high resolution CAT scan is usually made. If the scan is normal, as it often is, a decision about surgery will be greatly influenced by the finding of a consistent EEG abnormality, supported if necessary by sphenoidal lead tracings. The potentially good surgical results for highly selected children and adolescents justify such invasive investigation in special centres. The role of CAT scanning for children with epilepsy has been reviewed by Lagenstein et al. (1980).

The capacity to assay drug and metabolite levels in serum and saliva from children receiving anticonvulsant treatment has been a major advance. This enables compliance with treatment to be assessed and has also taught us much about the variation in individual responses to medication.

CONCLUSION

The natural history of epilepsies in childhood needs to be understood by those who treat affected children; investigation is planned in the light of such knowledge (Ounsted et al., 1966; Hauser et al., 1980; Okuma and Kumashiro, 1981; Sofijanov, 1982; Beghi et al., 1982). Both the affected children and their families need to understand the purpose and implication of such investigations if their full cooperation is to be obtained. It is the practice in our department to offer discussion with our informed social worker, as well as with the medical staff, to facilitate discussion of these issues.

REFERENCES

BAUMANN, R. J., MARX, M. B., and LEONIDAKIS, M. G. (1978) Epilepsy in rural Kentucky: prevalence in a population of school age children. *Epilepsia*, **19**, 75–80.

BEAUSSART, M. (1972) Benign epilepsy of children with rolandic (centro-temporal) paroxysmal foci. A clinical entity. Study of 221 cases. *Epilepsia*, **13**, 795–811.

BEGHI, E., SASANELLI, F., SPAGNOLI, A., and TOGNONI, G. (1982) Quality of care of epilepsy in Italy: a multi-hospital survey of diagnosis and treatment of 1104 epileptic patients. *Epilepsia*, **23**, 133–148.

BERNARDINA, B. D., and BEGHINI, G. (1976) Rolandic spikes in children with and without epilepsy (20 subjects polygraphically studied during sleep). *Epilepsia*, **17**, 161–167.

BRITISH MEDICAL JOURNAL (1979) Doubtful epilepsy in childhood. *Br. Med. J.*, **2**, 1–2.

CHEVRIE, J. J., and AICARDI, J. (1978) Convulsive disorders in the first year of life: Neurological and mental outcome and mortality. *Epilepsia*, **19**, 67–74.

EEG-OLOFSSON, O., PETERSEN, I., and SELLDEN, U. (1971) The development of the electroencephalogram in normal children from the age of 1 through 15 years. Paroxysmal activity. *Neuropaediatrie*, **2**, 375–404.

HAUSER, W. A., ANNEGERS, J. F., and ELVEBACK, L. R. (1980) Mortality in patients with epilepsy. *Epilepsia*, **21**, 399–412.

LAGENSTEIN, I., STERNOWSKY, H. J., ROTHE, M., BENTELE, K. H., and KÜHNE, G. (1980) CCT in different epilepsies with grand mal and focal seizures in 309 children: relation to clinical and electroencephalographic data. *Neuropediatrics*, **11**, 323–338.

LERMAN, P., and KIVITY-EPHRAIM, S. (1981) Focal epileptic EEG discharges in children not suffering from clinical epilepsy: etiology, clinical significance, and management. *Epilepsia*, **22**, 551–558.

OKUMA, T., and KUMASHIRO, H. (1981) Natural history and prognosis of epilepsy: report of a multi-institutional study in Japan. *Epilepsia*, **22**, 35–53.

OUNSTED, C., LINDSAY, J., and NORMAN, R. (1966) Biological factors in temporal lobe epilepsy. *Clinics in Developmental Medicine 22*. Medical Education and Information Unit, The Spastics Society, London. Heinemann, London.

SINGER, W. D., HALLER, J. S., SULLIVAN, J. R., WOLPERT, S., MILLS, C., and RABE, E. F. (1982) The value of neuroradiology in infantile spasms. *J. Pediatr.*, **100**, 47–50.

SOFIJANOV, N. G. (1982) Clinical evolution and prognosis of childhood epilepsies. *Epilepsia*, **23**, 61–69.

STORES, G. (1984) Intensive EEG monitoring in paediatrics. *Dev. Med. Child Neurol.*, **26**, 231–234.

Paediatric Perspectives on Epilepsy
Edited by E. Ross and E. Reynolds
© 1985 John Wiley & Sons Ltd.

14

Counselling the parent of the child with epilepsy*

STUART GREEN
Institute of Child Health, Birmingham

SUMMARY

The parents of children with epilepsy need to understand the nature of the terrifying and unpredictable paroxysms that suddenly take their children from them – and to know how best to handle them. Their children need to be kept in the picture and appropriately informed about their own condition. And the specialists, family doctor and others responsible need to be readily available, not simply to listen, to inform and to give advice, but to tailor that information and advice to individual needs.

A simple framework of questions covers the basic information that parents require: What is epilepsy? What causes it? What is the treatment? What is the follow-up? What is the effect on schooling? What restrictions are required? What is the duration of treatment? And what is the future? Parents can also be reassured that most children who are normal apart from their epilepsy are likely to have a good outcome, though the prospects are less hopeful in cases of refractory epilepsy.

INTRODUCTION

Many of the patients whom I see as a second opinion come to me not only because they have complex epilepsy but because their parents do not understand about the situation and would like some further explanation.

Why is it that parents need this information? Because epilepsy is such a terrifying disease. Its paroxysmal nature – the fact that the child is suddenly

*This chapter is an edited transcript of Stuart Green's contribution to the Eastbourne conference.

taken away, as it were, and sometimes appears to be dead – is what frightens parents. They need to know what epilepsy is, what causes it, how it is treated and followed up, its effects on schooling, the duration of treatment, what restrictions are necessary, and the prospects for the future.

WHAT IS EPILEPSY?

Many parents have terrible guilt about epilepsy, for which they feel responsible. It is very important to explain to people of all levels of sophistication that epilepsy is a physical disease, not psychiatric, not due to something done in early life, and not due to possession or evil malice. There are many misconceptions about epilepsy – including what people in the family have died of, and other diseases which appear to be similar. Parents need to be told that epilepsy does not necessarily mean that the child will become brain-damaged or develop abnormal behaviour, and that it is often perfectly compatible with a normal life.

What about the word 'epilepsy'? I think it is better that parents should hear the word epilepsy from me – rather than complain after many months: 'We thought it was only convulsions, but the lady next door said . . . Why didn't you tell us it was epilepsy?' When epilepsy has been established, it is better to say so, explaining that there are different types and that we will try to find the underlying cause.

WHAT IS THE CAUSE?

The concept of seed and soil is very helpful. Parents should be informed that there may be genetic predisposition or an underlying disease process of which epilepsy is a manifestation – despite the fact that, for some people, the diagnosis of epilepsy is all the more terrible because it means the uncovering of a serious underlying condition. Such a diagnosis is followed by the well-known reactions of anger, denial and then gradual acceptance. This needs very careful counselling. For others, diagnosis of epilepsy may actually come as a relief, because it explains a puzzling behavioural disturbance, for example. Investigations need to be clearly explained. We may think a normal result can wait until the next appointment, but the parents may be anxious to hear sooner. Some parents become extremely concerned about the results of CT scans: 'I knew you thought the child had a tumour otherwise you wouldn't have done a CT (cerebral tumour) scan, would you?' Worries of this kind can be countered at the outset by saying that the vast majority of children with epilepsy do not have a tumour. The idea that they do is still very widespread.

Depending on the age and sophistication of the child, he or she should be told why the attacks occur and what epilepsy is. Some variation of Hughlings Jackson's original definition – about an occasional, disorderly discharge of nerve tissue – can be very helpful, perhaps likening it to an abnormal electrical discharge or to some sort of daydream or funny turn.

HOW IS IT TREATED?

First, I explain to parents that the management is for the most part going to be long-term. Otherwise some may think that a single course of treatment is all that the child needs – as with pneumonia or meningitis. Even when anticonvulsant therapy is short-term or not necessary at all, there is still likely to be a need for long-term follow-up. Whenever treatment is given, it is very important to explain that the drugs must be taken regularly. Both the parents and, if possible, the patient *must* know the drugs they are prescribed, and the dosage. Since many people may be involved in the management of a child with epilepsy, it is very useful to give the parents a card on which all changes in treatment are recorded. The same card can also be used to record any seizures that occur. One parent said: 'I thought what I wanted from you was information. Now I realize that what's needed is an *exchange* of information'. Unless you tell them, the parents may not realize that you need information from them about what is going on.

Parents and patients also need information about what to do in emergencies. This is well described in many handouts and books (see page 121) which parents of children with epilepsy find valuable as sources of background information. The support of self-help associations can also be of major assistance: some addresses are given overleaf.

WHAT IS THE FOLLOW-UP?

My personal practice is to carry on with management of the children until the diagnosis is clearly established, and explained, and some degree of control initiated. Depending on the original referral, I then refer the child back to the paediatrician or, occasionally, to the general practitioner. Rightly or wrongly, I follow up many of the patients myself. Whoever is responsible, there *must* be a lifeline between the parents and the doctor for cases of difficulty (not necessarily emergencies) regarding behaviour, schooling and changes in drug therapy. A team approach, perhaps with a nurse or social worker, can extend this information gathering and sharing. People do feel a need for some sort of continuous link.

WHAT IS THE EFFECT ON SCHOOLING?

Most children with epilepsy go to normal schools, and I take it upon myself to communicate with the school doctor as necessary, and ensure that the school is properly informed. Behavioural and cognitive problems have already been touched upon, but one thing I try and explain to parents is that there may be no simple answers to these very difficult problems if there is underlying brain disease. And in every case we have to consider the possible effects not only of the epilepsy itself, associated with actual and/or subclinical seizures, but also of anticonvulsant therapy. There may be very complex interactions, and we should be very careful not to attribute any deterioration or change in behaviour to one particular factor. It is very rarely possible to pinpoint the cause of behavioural problems without taking a global view, and the doctor should be in a good position to receive information from the parents, the school, the school doctor and others, and then to consider, together with the parents, what can be done to try and break the cycle of deterioration – perhaps by a change in drugs or dosage, perhaps by changing the school, perhaps by counselling the parents. This is a most difficult area.

WHAT RESTRICTIONS ARE NECESSARY?

This is always a controversial topic, but there are a few things which I think ought to be observed in all children with epilepsy. Obviously these restrictions are going to vary with intellectual capacity, behaviour, and type of seizure. The dangers affecting all epileptic children that are most important to mention include: fire, swimming, cycling and climbing. Children whose epilepsy is not well controlled are much more prone to burns, and *all* fires – open and electric – must be guarded. As regards swimming, I see no reason why otherwise normal children with epilepsy, and even many retarded or cerebral palsy children with epilepsy, should not go swimming *as long as they are supervised*. If the school cannot do this, the parents should be encouraged to go to the school and swim with the child, or the American 'buddy system' should be adopted, to make an older child responsible. Some people suggest that this should be done anyway as a precaution. There is then very little reason why the vast majority of children with epilepsy should not swim.

Cycling in traffic is somewhat dangerous anyway, but for those children who have drop attacks or sudden loss of consciousness without warning it should be done only under the closest supervision. There is seldom need to restrict ordinary PT or games, but sudden seizures at the top of a rope can obviously be dangerous. Competitive games, even those involving stress or anxiety, should not generally be prescribed. Indeed, there is a danger that the possibility of stress and anxiety provoking seizures may become the focus of management. It is better for the child to be encouraged to live as normal a life as possible.

WHAT IS THE DURATION OF TREATMENT?

With children who are otherwise normal, there is a good chance – perhaps about 80% – that they will be able to come off anticonvulsant drugs in a few years if the seizures are controlled. I tell parents this at an early stage, stressing the need for regular treatment meanwhile, and pointing out that it is better for some children to continue treatment, and thus be free of seizures, than to be off drugs.

With refractory epilepsy, one has to explain that it may not be possible to achieve good control, and that increasing the drugs is going to make the child more sedated – adversely affecting school work and perhaps behaviour. Some parents accept such compromises more readily than others.

WHAT IS THE FUTURE?

Most children who are otherwise normal are likely to have a good outcome. In such cases, I like to emphasize to the children themselves that many people in adult life are epileptic and yet live normal lives – growing up, going to university, studying, getting married and having children. Obviously this does not apply to those with refractory epilepsy. Perhaps the best approach for them is to adopt the old philosophy of curing sometimes, modifying often, but always supporting the families and parents of children with epilepsy. Maybe this is the software of epilepsy management, but, as with computers, it is the software that makes the hardware run smoothly.

INFORMATION ON EPILEPSY FOR FAMILIES

*BERAN, R. G. (1982) *Learning about Epilepsy.* Medical Education (Services) Ltd., Oxford.

LAIDLAW, M. V., and LAIDLAW, J. (1980) *Epilepsy Explained.* Churchill Livingstone, Edinburgh.

LAGOS, J. C. (1974) *Epilepsy and Your Child. A Handbook for Parents, Teachers and Epileptics of All Ages.* Harper and Row, London.

McGOVERN, S. (1982) *The Epilepsy Handbook.* Sheldon Press, London.

O'DONOHOE, N. V. (1975–1977) *Epilepsy Today. Epilepsy in Childhood.* Geigy Pharmaceuticals, Horsham. (Compiled from: *Epilepsy Today – Management Guidelines for the Practitioner. Growing Points in Childhood Epilepsy*, Parts 1–5. Geigy Pharmaceuticals, Macclesfield, 1975–1977.)

*YOUNG, H. (1980) *What Difference Does it Make, Danny?* André Deutsch, London.

*For children themselves

SOCIETIES

British Epilepsy Association   Tel. 0344 773122
Crowthorne House
New Wokingham Road
WOKINGHAM
Berks RG11 3AY
(Offices also in Birmingham, Leeds, Belfast and Cardiff)

'In Touch'   Tel. 061 962 4441
Mrs Ann Worthington
10 Norman Road
SALE
Cheshire M33 3DF

Discussion

Dr S. Rose (Inverness): You have given us a lot of information about counselling, Dr Green, and your approach came across as paternalistic. Of the information you give to the parents – presumably over a period of time – can you say how much is totally misconstrued, or misunderstood, or indeed retained?

Green: I do not at the moment have such information, but I agree that monitoring is needed. I am hoping to have working with me somebody like a health visitor or counsellor who will be available to consider some of these aspects. We are going to compare two inner districts to try and analyse the difference over a period of time in patients' response and understanding. I do not know whether patients retain what I say, but some of them do say at the time that this is the first time they have had an explanation of what has been going on, and they appear to understand. Sometimes what I say may cause anxiety, but in some situations you have to upset people so that they understand. When I see patients a second or third time and they still have not understood what is happening, then it becomes obvious I failed them the first time. That is why I have stressed the need to modify management according to each patient's degree of sophistication. Some immigrant families who come from the simplest backgrounds have been plucked from a mediaeval culture and plonked in 20th century Birmingham. Yes, to some extent I am paternalistic, although that is changing as people become more sophisticated and ask more questions.

Dr B. Mason (Worcester): I look after a fairly sophisticated population, but I would say that most of my patients who see Dr Green remember most of what he says. A question that concerns me is how we can influence schools. Usually there is an approachable teacher, headmistress or headmaster, but there does not seem to be any mechanism to get doctors and actual class teachers together.

Green: Working in a regional centre, I deal with 22 different districts each of which has a school medical service organized in a different way. I do my best to communicate with the appropriate school medical officer. I think that should be my channel of communication. The problem is, he or she does not necessarily communicate well with the school, and the head teacher who has the relevant information does not communicate with the teacher. Where there are special problems, I ask the parents if they have any objection to my telling the teacher. Few parents object to a teacher being told of the child's problem if they feel it is going to help.

Dr B. D. Bower (Oxford): If Stuart Green is thought to be paternalistic, then I must be thought to be grandpaternalistic. In our clinic we have a part-time social worker, female, who is a lot younger than me and therefore closer to the family, with whom I have a rather different relationship. Many misconceptions are sorted out between them, initially and on subsequent occasions, both at clinic attendances and also on the telephone. Perhaps not everybody can achieve this, but it is useful if you can.

Secondly, I have a question about fishing. In my area boys want to go fishing by themselves – it is not the same if they fish in company. Some of them are extremely keen, and go off very early in the morning on this solitary activity, sitting on a river bank. What do you feel my response should be?

Green: I have never been asked that question, but if a child wanted very much to go fishing I would say you have to take the risk. I have never absolutely stopped a child doing what he wanted, except on one occasion. This was an eight-year-old who had flicker-induced photosensitive generalized epilepsy and rode motor bikes – scrambling in the summer through dappled trees in the country. The parents refused to stop that, and I regretted that I could not continue treatment in that situation. In general, we must allow reasonable risks in life, especially if the child is sensible.

Dr A. J. Franklin (Chelmsford): It is my impression that the greatest stress in schools comes from other schoolchildren. Have you any thoughts about that?

Green: In all handicap, children are often cruel to other children. One of the reasons I use the word epilepsy, perhaps more frequently than some of my paediatric colleagues, is that I want, as it were, to 'detoxify' the word.

Eeg-Olofsson: In young schoolchildren stress-induced seizures are not very common, but become more frequent around puberty and adolescence. The first information given to children and their parents is extremely important in such cases.

Ross: I believe there is a need for a children's epilepsy clinic in each district. With the gradual transformation of child health to a consultant-led service, both hospital and community based, there is some prospect of moving towards this aim. Whether an epilepsy clinic should be named as such or called a children's handicap or child neurology clinic is largely a matter of taste. In the district of Brent, in North London, we ran a children's epilepsy clinic, under that name. Market research showed that about 85% of parents liked the fact that the word epilepsy was used and not some euphemism. On the other hand, quite a lot of children who came to this clinic did not actually have epilepsy.

Dr M. R. Trimble (London): In our clinic at Queen Square we were looking for the right paramedical person to help us and chose the sister on our ward. At first the nursing authorities were a bit hesitant but then saw that this was a good idea – and feasible for one afternoon a week. We tried to give her some special tutoring in epilepsy, and her presence at the clinic had two main benefits. First, many outpatients knew her after discharge from the ward. Second, she could tell the patients when she would be on the ward, so they had a hotline to somebody they knew. The disappointing part was that many adult patients wanted to talk to her about their marital and financial difficulties rather than about their epilepsy, which they still wanted to discuss with the doctor.

My question to Dr Green is this: Who do you think is the most appropriate paramedical person to have working with you in a clinic?

Green: Particularly for young children, I think somebody with nursing experience is important, coupled with health visitor training and, ideally, experience as a school nurse.

If she has an interest in psychology and behaviour, so much the better. I am waiting for this ideal person to turn up.

Eeg-Olofsson: In Sweden we have a nurse with experience in psychology and social problems, to work not only with epilepsy but also with allergy and diabetes in childhood.

McKinlay: In Manchester our department meets on Monday mornings to plan the week's work, to discuss present and future inpatients, and to explain the purpose of the admission. Our ward social worker is present at that meeting. She then offers an appointment to each inpatient's family during the admission and follows that up after discharge. A social worker who has been in the department for some time, has learnt about the sort of work we are doing, and had it explained over a period of time, is perfectly well able to fulfil the role that we are discussing. I do not think it matters too much which profession paramedics come from, so long as they are party to the medical plans and discussion and able to translate that to families – and also to translate what families say back to us.

Dr M. J. Noronha (Manchester): The point Dr Green made about telling parents that we have reached the end of the road in controlling their child's seizures is very important. As clinicians, we have to know our own limitations. But, on the question of restrictions for children with epilepsy, I would hate to see the children I am treating go riding their bikes on the road. While looking to their welfare, we have also to consider the welfare of the general public.

Green: If a child has just started learning to ride a bike and is excited by it and gets a few seizures, it is going to be a terrible disappointment to him to stop him riding the bike. I think we should strike a balance. We should certainly be very careful about riding in busy traffic, but riding in a park or side streets may be acceptable. There is a borderline, and much depends on where you live. In Birmingham or Manchester it is madness to ride a bike anyway.

Dr P. N. Christie (Kingston): Particularly for children with more severe handicap, the person who can often do a great deal is the class teacher backed by the head teacher. I have a policy of actually going into the school, often meeting with the parents and other people involved with the child. Some children see more of their teachers than of their parents at certain times in their lives. Teachers can also help monitor the management of the more severely handicapped children.

Paediatric Perspectives on Epilepsy
Edited by E. Ross and E. Reynolds
© 1985 John Wiley & Sons Ltd.

15

Treatment of the schoolchild with epilepsy

Breege M. MacArdle
*Department of Paediatric Neurology, Guy's Hospital, London, and
Department of Child Health, King's College Hospital, London*

SUMMARY

Anticonvulsant drug therapy for most schoolchildren with epilepsy should be started after two afebrile seizures, provided that the diagnosis can be confirmed. In high-risk cases, treatment may be indicated after a single seizure. The anticonvulsant to be given depends on the seizure type and on the individual patient's response to therapy. Initial dosage should be low. In most schoolchildren with epilepsy the seizures can be controlled by monotherapy with one of the three major anticonvulsants – phenytoin, carbamazepine or sodium valproate – at increased dosage if necessary. If seizures cannot be controlled with monotherapy, a second anticonvulsant drug may need to be added. Treatment should generally be continued until the child has been free of seizures on treatment for four years – and withdrawal should always be slow.

INTRODUCTION

Epilepsy is a common problem in paediatric practice; about five per thousand children of school age have recurrent afebrile seizures (Ross *et al.*, 1980). The indications for commencing anticonvulsant therapy, the choice of drug and duration of treatment in the schoolchild with epilepsy will be reviewed. Before undertaking the commitment of long-term anticonvulsant medication, the physician must be quite confident of the diagnosis. A witness account is of vital importance, although in some cases even the parents' history should be doubted (Meadow, 1984).

Of 201 children with a possible diagnosis of epilepsy newly referred to a paediatric clinic, there was definite doubt about the diagnosis in nearly 50% and in three-quarters of these the attacks proved to be non-epileptic (Robinson, 1984).

INDICATIONS FOR COMMENCING ANTICONVULSANT THERAPY

Many children are referred to hospital following a single seizure. Should we suggest commencing therapy at this stage? A small number of studies in children have been carried out attempting to answer this question. The quoted risk of subsequent seizures varies from 5% (Costeff and Avni, 1982) to 27% (Hauser et al., 1982), and can be as high as 90% (Livingston, 1958). Interpretation of these studies is confounded by a lack of information on some patients, by inclusion of acute neurological disease and by the fact that many patients were started on therapy after their first seizure. However, certain factors seem to be associated with a higher recurrence rate (Table I). There is some evidence

Table I   Factors which increase the risk of subsequent afebrile seizures

Previous neurological insult[1,2]
Absence attacks (three per second spike and wave)[1]
Benign focal epilepsy[2]
Positive family history[2]

[1]Blom et al., 1978.
[2]Hauser et al., 1982.

that early treatment of seizures improves prognosis (Shorvon and Reynolds, 1982). One should seriously consider treating children in the high-risk group after their first seizure. In most cases treatment can be delayed until after the second seizure.

WHICH DRUGS SHOULD BE PRESCRIBED?

The goal of therapy is to prevent seizures with a minimum of side effects. The choice of drug should be based on seizure type. Many clinicians have their own preference.

In our prospective study of monotherapy in children, four major anti-convulsants have been compared – phenobarbitone, phenytoin, carbamazepine and sodium valproate – starting at low dosage and increasing as necessary. Among the 99 newly-diagnosed children with epilepsy so far studied the following points have emerged (McGowan et al., 1983; MacArdle et al., 1984). There is clearly a place for monotherapy in childhood epilepsy, the failure rate on monotherapy being 17%, which is similar to that in adult studies

(Shorvon *et al.*, 1978). Sodium valproate appears less effective in controlling partial seizures. Drug toxicity has not been a major problem, apart from behavioural side effects with phenobarbitone (which we have now stopped prescribing). About 25% of the children were withdrawn from our study,

Table II   Withdrawals from study of 99
children with epilepsy

Drug side effects	13
Adverse media coverage	2
Fatal overdose	1
Poor compliance	1
Lost to follow-up	2
Stopped drug	1
Fit free for two years	2
Total	22

illustrating some of the practical difficulties in caring for children with epilepsy (Table II). Clearly it is not yet possible to draw any firm conclusions about the efficacy of the major anticonvulsants; our numbers are small and the follow-up period is still relatively short (16 months).

HOW LONG SHOULD TREATMENT BE CONTINUED?

The overall outcome for childhood-onset epilepsy is good. The relapse rate after withdrawal of treatment, following a four-year period of freedom from seizures, is about 30% (Holowach *et al.*, 1972; Thurston *et al.*, 1982; Emerson *et al.*, 1981).

Patients whose epilepsy occurs between the ages of two and 16 years, with a small number of generalized seizures, without neurological or psychiatric handicap and whose EEG is normal, have a higher chance of remaining seizure free off treatment. A high number of seizures prior to remission is associated with a greater relapse rate. There is some controversy about the influence of the following factors on relapse: the presence of neurological dysfunction or mental retardation, and combinations of seizure types. It seems sensible to attempt withdrawal of therapy in most children who have been seizure free for four years, particularly as there is some concern about the susceptibility of retarded patients to cognitive side effects of drugs (Trimble, 1979). The rate of anticonvulsant withdrawal may also influence the subsequent relapse rate (Chadwick, 1984), and very slow withdrawal may improve the outlook. A multicentre study is currently being conducted in the UK to investigate the latter question and also withdrawal of therapy after two years' freedom from seizures.

CONCLUSION

The outlook for the majority of schoolchildren with epilepsy is excellent. There is probably no great difference in efficacy between the major anticonvulsants. The longer the child remains seizure free on therapy the greater the chance of long-term cure.

We have all been made aware of the importance of counselling and education of families and school teachers who have responsibility for children with epilepsy. Such an approach may help with the earlier identification of families at risk of developing significant problems.

REFERENCES

BLOM, S., HIEJBEL, J., and BERGFORS, P. G. (1978) Incidence of epilepsy in children: A follow-up study three years after the first seizure. *Epilepsia*, **19**, 343–350.

CHADWICK, D. (1984) The discontinuance of antiepileptic therapy. In: *Recent Advances in Epilepsy*, pp. 111–124 (Eds T. A. Pedley and B. S. Meldrum). Churchill Livingstone, Edinburgh.

COSTEFF, H., and AVNI, A. (1982) Reported seizures in early childhood: A 14-year follow-up. *Dev. Med. Child Neurol.*, **24**, 472–478.

EMERSON, R., D'SOUZA, B. J., VINING, E. P., HOLDEN, K. R., MELLITS, E. D., and FREEMAN, J. M. (1981) Stopping medication in children with epilepsy. *N. Engl. J. Med.*, **304**, 1125–1129.

HAUSER, W. A., ELVING ANDERSON, V., LOEWENSON, R. B., and MCROBERTS, S. M. (1982) Seizure recurrence after a first unprovoked seizure. *N. Engl. J. Med.*, **307**, 522–528.

HOLOWACH, J., THURSTON, D., and O'LEARY, J. (1972) Prognosis in childhood epilepsy. Follow-up study of 148 cases in which therapy has been suspended after prolonged anticonvulsant control. *N. Engl. J. Med.*, **286**, 169–174.

LIVINGSTON, S. (1958) Convulsive disorders in infants and children. *Adv. Pediatr.*, **10**, 113–195.

MACARDLE, B. M., MCGOWAN, M., JOHNSON, A. L., NEVILLE, B., and REYNOLDS, E. H. (1984) Randomized comparative trial of monotherapy in epileptic children. *Acta Neurol. Scand.*, **70**, 241.

MCGOWAN, M. E. L., NEVILLE, B. G. R., and REYNOLDS, E. H. (1983) Comparative monotherapy trial in children with epilepsy. *Br. J. Clin. Prac.*, **27** (Suppl.), 115–118.

MEADOW, R. (1984) Factitious illness – the hinterland of child abuse. In: *Recent Advances in Paediatrics*, 7, pp. 217–232 (Ed. R. Meadow). Churchill Livingstone, Edinburgh.

ROBINSON, R. J. (1984) When to start and stop anticonvulsants. In: *Recent Advances in Paediatrics*, 7, pp. 155–174 (Ed. R. Meadow). Churchill Livingstone, Edinburgh.

ROSS, E. M., PECKHAM, C. S., WEST, P. B., and BUTLER, N. R. (1980) Epilepsy in childhood; findings from the National Child Development Study. *Br. Med. J.*, **1**, 207–210.

SHORVON, S. D., CHADWICK, D., GALBRAITH, A. W., and REYNOLDS, E. H. (1978) One drug for epilepsy. *Br. Med. J.*, **1**, 474–476.

SHORVON, S. D., CHADWICK, D., GALBRAITH, A. W., and REYNOLDS, E. H. (1978) One drug for epilepsy. *Br. Med. J.*, **1**, 474–476.
SHORVON, S. D., and REYNOLDS, E. H. (1982) Early prognosis of epilepsy. *Br. Med. J.*, **285**, 1699–1701.
THURSTON, J., THURSTON, D., HIXON, B., and KELLER, A. (1982) Prognosis in childhood epilepsy. Additional follow-up of 148 children 15 to 23 years after withdrawal of anticonvulsant therapy. *N. Engl. J. Med.*, **306**, 831–836.
TRIMBLE, M. (1979) The effects of anticonvulsant drugs on cognitive abilities. *Pharmacol. Ther.*, **4**, 677–685.

Paediatric Perspectives on Epilepsy
Edited by E. Ross and E. Reynolds
© 1985 John Wiley & Sons Ltd.

16

Longitudinal studies of children's epilepsy

C. M. VERITY[1] (1970 cohort) and E. M. ROSS[2] (1958 cohort)
[1]*Bristol Royal Hospital for Sick Children, Bristol, and*
[2]*Charing Cross Hospital and Charing Cross and Westminster Medical School,
London*

SUMMARY

Prospective longitudinal studies provide a major source of information about
the frequency, nature and evolving patterns of childhood epilepsy.

The United Kingdom is unique in having carried out three such follow-up
studies of child development based on one-week birth cohorts, starting in 1946,
1958 and 1970. Comparing the findings obtained in the 1958 and 1970 cohorts,
there has been little change in the overall prevalence of seizure disorders or
in frequency of febrile convulsions, despite major improvements in perinatal
care. And the National Child Development Study (of the 1958 cohort) found
that about 70% of epilepsy was primary, leaving relatively little scope for
prevention. The majority of children with seizure disorders do well, however,
both intellectually and in tending to 'grow out of' their epilepsy.

INTRODUCTION

A full understanding of the problem of childhood epilepsy can only be achieved
by studying its evolution during childhood development. Knowledge of health
prior to the seizure is vital, but few doctors can follow large numbers of children
for long periods. Much published work comes from hospitals that treat only
the worst cases, and children with less severe attacks or spontaneous remission
of epilepsy may never be studied.

The United Kingdom is unique in having carried out three longitudinal studies
of child development based on one-week cohorts of children born in 1946

(Cooper, 1965), 1958 (Ross *et al.*, 1980) and 1970 (Chamberlain *et al.*, 1975). In each of these years all infants born in a selected spring week were studied in detail from birth. Their subsequent progress has formed a useful basis for learning about epilepsy in unselected children, and in this paper the findings from the 1958 and 1970 cohorts are discussed.

FOLLOW-UP STUDIES

The National Child Development Study (NCDS)

This included all children born in one week in March 1958, aiming to trace them to their schools at ages seven, 11 and 16 and to their homes at 23. On the first three occasions about 90% were contacted: health visitors interviewed parents at home, school doctors took medical histories and performed examinations, school teachers completed educational ratings and administered educational tests. At 23, the young adults were interviewed by market research field workers. A special substudy of children with epilepsy was set up soon after the 11-year follow-up had been completed. By this stage 1043 of the 15 496 children for whom information had been gathered at seven and 11 years had a record suggestive of at least one fit, faint or turn. Further information on these 1043 children was obtained by means of a postal questionnaire, epilepsy being defined as 'recurrent paroxysmal disturbance of consciousness, sensation or movement, primarily cerebral in origin, unassociated with acute febrile episodes'. The children finally regarded as having epilepsy were then reviewed at the subsequent follow-ups at 16 and 23 years of age.

The Child Health and Education Study (CHES)

This started as the 'British Births Survey', which studied all the children born in one week in April 1970. Full details about the mother, the pregnancy, labour, delivery and first postpartum week were obtained by midwives. Survivors living in Great Britain were seen at home when they were five years old. Local health visitors completed detailed questionnaires about the medical history and social background of the children. They also administered tests of performance. Of the 13 135 children seen at five years of age, 767 had a history suggestive of at least one seizure. Further information about these children was obtained by means of a questionnaire sent to general practitioners (87% reply rate) and by borrowing the hospital notes for study (97% of the notes were obtained). It was then possible to reach a conclusion as to the nature of the episode of disturbed consciousness in the majority of the children in whom such an episode had been reported. This could be correlated with the information already available on all the children, enabling those with a history of seizures to be compared with the rest of the study population.

FINDINGS

Seizures in the first week

The British Births Survey revealed that 72 children (0.4%) had one or more 'fits or convulsions' during the first week of life (Chamberlain *et al.*, 1975). There was a dramatic increase in the mortality rate among babies with cerebral irritability who developed fits. This was particularly marked in the low-birthweight babies (Fig. 1). Of all the babies with first-week fits 15 died – an overall mortality rate of 21%, much greater than the 0.9% mortality rate in those with cerebral irritation but no fits.

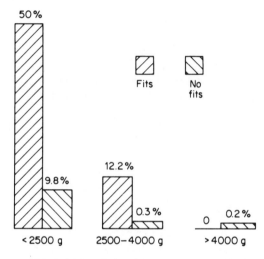

Fig. 1 1970 British Births Survey. Babies with cerebral irritation: percentage mortality rate in three different birth-weight groups according to the presence or absence of fits

Febrile convulsions

Febrile convulsions occur before children are five years old. Figure 2 (from a previous report of CHES findings) shows that more than 60% of children have their first fit by the age of two years. When they were studied at five years of age, 2.2% of the CHES children had suffered from febrile convulsions, 64% of these having had only one attack. By seven years, 2.4% of NCDS children had suffered from febrile convulsions, two-thirds of them having had a single attack. The proportion admitted to hospital rose from 45% in the NCDS to 61% in the CHES study; of these, one third had a lumbar puncture, the majority on the first admission. Neither study found much influence of perinatal events

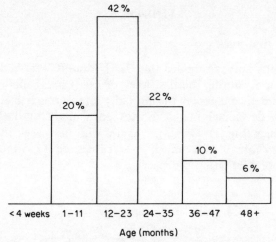

Fig. 2   CHES data. Age of onset of febrile convulsions:
percentage of total group having their first attack at the ages
shown (from Golding and Butler, 1983)

on the subsequent development of febrile convulsions, or much variation in
incidence between the social classes, but both found a slight excess of boys.

These studies can also help to answer some important questions about febrile
convulsions. Do they 'cause' later epilepsy? Alternatively, are a significant
number of truly epileptic children initially misdiagnosed as suffering from febrile
convulsions because their temperature and other details of the attack are
inadequately documented? The NCDS data show that a small minority of
children with febrile convulsions are eventually diagnosed as epileptic, the rate
being only 0.5% in those managed entirely at home. The rate increases to 15%
among children admitted to hospital for febrile convulsions, giving an overall
rate of 5%. This information suggests two things. First, it might be expected
that children managed at home would be more prone to misdiagnosis than those
admitted to hospital, where documentation is more complete. If misdiagnosis
contributes significantly to the occurrence of epilepsy after an initial supposedly
febrile convulsion, a higher rate of eventual epilepsy would therefore be found
among those children managed at home – the reverse of what was actually found.
The NCDS is therefore against the 'misdiagnosis' theory. Second, it seems likely
that the children with more severe attacks are admitted to hospital and that
they are at greater risk of developing later epilepsy. The CHES data tend to
confirm the supposition that the more severe cases are admitted to hospital – a
greater proportion of children with 'complex' febrile convulsions (focal, repeated
or prolonged) were admitted than with 'simple' attacks.

The data at present available from NCDS and CHES thus indicate a
reassuringly low rate of epilepsy after febrile convulsions, but the risk is greater
in those children with more severe attacks. Similar findings were reported by

Nelson and Ellenberg (1976) in their analysis of the data yielded by the large Collaborative Perinatal Project in the United States: epilepsy developed by seven years of age in 1.5% of otherwise normal children with 'non-complex' first febrile seizures, as opposed to 4.1% of children with complex first febrile seizures. Febrile convulsions may in themselves be responsible for some of the later afebrile attacks. Alternatively, the same pre-existing neurological abnormality could be responsible for both febrile and afebrile attacks in those children later diagnosed as epileptic. Neither the NCDS nor the CHES yield data which enable us to decide which of these alternatives is correct.

There is another important question: do children who have had febrile convulsions show behavioural or intellectual deficits as they grow up? Even without physical damage, the parental alarm engendered by the attacks might lead to differences in the way parents relate to their children. Happily, the CHES findings at five years show no significant differences in behaviour or attainment between the febrile-convulsion children and the rest. The NCDS follow-up to 11 years showed no emerging pattern of deficit. Neither study has found evidence that febrile convulsions in themselves lead to cerebral dysfunction. The CHES data showed that the 13 children known to have a neurological abnormality preceding the first febrile convulsion did significantly less well on tests of performance than the rest of the cohort. Such patients have been included in some previous studies of progress after febrile convulsions and this may well have led to reports of poor outcome. Ellenberg and Nelson (1978) have reported on the good prognosis for intellectual performance after febrile seizures.

Non-febrile epilepsy and school progress

By the age of five years, 38 children in the CHES (2.9 per 1000) had a history of at least one afebrile primary generalized seizure. Since epilepsy is conventionally regarded as a recurrent seizure disorder, it is not possible to quote the true prevalence at this stage. By age seven, 34 children in the NCDS (2.2 per 1000) had had at least two afebrile seizures and were regarded as having epilepsy. Table I shows the diagnostic categories of NCDS children with reported fits, based on information obtained at seven or 11, or both. There is, however, controversy as to which children should be regarded as having epilepsy; for example, should seizures in early infancy be discounted? If all children who ever had a generalized afebrile seizure (including secondary or symptomatic attacks) are included, the proportion of the CHES cohort with attacks rises to 7.8 per 1000 by the age of five.

The NCDS showed that by age 11 a total of 103 children were regarded by at least one of their professional advisers as 'having epilepsy'. In 39 cases this diagnosis was not thought to be tenable in the light of available information, leaving 64 with clear-cut epilepsy (4.1 per 1000). The children could be divided into two main groups – two-thirds being educated solely in the normal

Table I   National Child Development Study: Diagnostic categories of children with reported fits; information from seven and/or 11 years of age from total number of study children (15 496)

Category	Children affected	
	Number	Per 1000
'Definite' epilepsy	64	4.1
'Epilepsy' reported by doctor but unsubstantiated	39	2.5
Febrile convulsions without later afebrile seizures	346	22.3
Febrile convulsions with later spontaneous afebrile seizures	20	1.3
Convulsions with meningitis or encephalitis	12	0.8
Breath-holding attacks Faints without convulsions Temper tantrums	280	18.1
Non-epileptic blank spells (confirmed by general practitioner or hospital)	7	0.5
Transitory afebrile convulsive episode not occurring after age 5 years	307	20.6
Convulsions reported by parent but not to general practitioner or hospital	12	0.8

educational system, the rest receiving special education. The former tended to have primary generalized epilepsy, and the majority of them had no seizures between 14 and 16 years of age. Their abilities measured by standardized tests of reading and maths at age 16 were below, but within one standard deviation of, the mean score for the study – indicating that a child with epilepsy who had the ability to remain in a normal school had good prospects of reasonable academic achievement and cessation of seizures. A much gloomier picture emerged among children in special education – 59% were still having fits in their 16th year and only three were regarded as able to cope with everyday reading needs. Only three of the 21 children were assessed as being in special need of educational placement because of their epilepsy – most were in special education because of intellectual deficit.

CONCLUSIONS

The NCDS and CHES findings are similar in many respects, despite differences in design between the two studies. The prevalence of febrile convulsions is very similar in the two studies, and there is little evidence that seizure disorders have become any less common in the 12 years separating the studies. Although perinatal care improved greatly between the studies, there is little evidence even in 1958 that perinatal problems were responsible for later seizures. The NCDS found that about 70% of epilepsy was primary, leaving relatively little scope for prevention in our present state of knowledge.

Longitudinal studies reveal the changing pattern of seizure disorders in childhood. The majority do well, both in terms of their eventual intellectual outcome and their tendency to 'grow out of' their disorders. There is a need to continue the follow-up for as long as possible so that we can see what the long-term outlook for childhood epilepsy really is. There is also a strong case for further national cohort studies; unfortunately the 12-year cycle has already been broken, and no time should be wasted if the expertise required to set up these studies is not to be lost.

ACKNOWLEDGEMENTS

Both studies spring from the genius of Professor Neville Butler, in Bristol, who generated the enthusiasm that created them out of the original birth-week studies. The 1958-based NCDS is currently directed by Dr R. Davie at the National Children's Bureau, London. The epilepsy substudy was initially funded by the Epilepsy Research Fund of the British Epilepsy Association and currently by Action Research for the Crippled Child. The work was originally carried out in Bristol, in collaboration with Dr Patrick West, and later in Charing Cross and Middlesex Hospital Medical Schools, in collaboration with Dr Catherine Peckham.

The 1970 births were followed up by the Child Health and Education Study at Bristol University in collaboration with Dr Jean Golding. The parent studies were funded from a variety of sources – governmental and charitable. Both studies were dependent on the unstinting help of large numbers of young people, their parents, school teachers, health visitors and doctors.

REFERENCES

CHAMBERLAIN, R., CHAMBERLAIN, G., HOWLETT, B., and CLAIREAUX, A. (1975) *British Births 1970. Volume I: The First Week of Life*, pp. 122–130. Heinemann, London.

COOPER, J. E. (1965) Epilepsy in a longitudinal study of 5000 children. *Br. Med. J.*, 1, 1020–1022.

ELLENBERG, J. H., and NELSON, K. B. (1978) Febrile seizures and later intellectual performance. *Arch. Neurol.*, 35, 17–21.

GOLDING, J., and BUTLER, N. R. (1983) Convulsive disorders in the Child Health and Education Study. In: *Research Progress in Epilepsy*, pp. 60–70 (Ed. F. C. Rose). Pitman, London.

NELSON, K. B., and ELLENBERG, J. H. (1976) Predictors of epilepsy in children who have experienced febrile seizures. *N. Engl. J. Med.*, **295**, 1029–1033.

ROSS, E. M., PECKHAM, C. S., WEST, P. B., and BUTLER, N. R. (1980) Epilepsy in childhood: findings from the National Child Development Study. *Br. Med. J.*, **1**, 207–210.

VERITY, C. M., BUTLER, N. R., and GOLDING, J. (1985) Febrile convulsions in a national cohort followed up from birth. *Br. Med. J.*, **1**, 1307–1315.

Paediatric Perspectives on Epilepsy
Edited by E. Ross and E. Reynolds
© 1985 John Wiley & Sons Ltd

17

Anticonvulsant drugs, cognitive function and behaviour

MICHAEL R. TRIMBLE[1,2] and PAMELA J. THOMPSON[1,3]
[1]*National Hospitals for Nervous Diseases and*
[2]*Institute of Neurology, Queen Square, London, and*
[3]*Chalfont Centre for Epilepsy, Gerrards Cross, Bucks*

SUMMARY

Impairment of cognitive function and behaviour can occur in association with epilepsy, and it has been suggested that anticonvulsant treatment may sometimes be related to this. To throw further light on the problem, studies have been made of a large population of children with epilepsy resident in a hospital school. A significant percentage of these children, given intelligence tests repeated after not less than one year, showed deterioration in IQ by more than 15 points; these children had serum levels of phenytoin and primidone significantly higher than the rest of the population. As regards behaviour, 50% of children receiving phenobarbitone were rated as having conduct disorder. When serum levels were examined, a negative correlation between carbamazepine levels and conduct disorder was noted.

Differences between anticonvulsant drugs in relation to cognitive function have also been seen in studies with adults. In these, patients had their cognitive state monitored while undergoing changes in anticonvulsant drug prescription. In one study, polytherapy has been rationalized; in two others, one with patients on monotherapy, patients have been tested at high and low serum levels. From these studies it is concluded that phenytoin impairs cognitive function, the effect being dose-dependent. Sodium valproate has less effect, although again this is dose dependent. Carbamazepine provokes minimal impairment and sometimes even improves scores. From other studies it is concluded that carbamazepine has mood-stabilizing properties, and is as effective as major tranquillizers in controlling acute mania.

INTRODUCTION

Chronic toxic effects of anticonvulsant drugs have been recognized for many years, but only recently has their impact on both cognitive function and behaviour become an area of interest. While not all cognitive or behavioural impairment in epilepsy can be attributed to drugs (hereditary, degenerative disorders, brain injury antedating seizures, psychological handicaps and epilepsy *per se* are among the causes listed by Lennox), the possibility that they contribute to it has been suggested for a number of years. One of the difficulties in assigning side effects has been the length of time for some of the chronic toxic effects of anticonvulsants to be recognized, following introduction of the drug to clinical practice (Reynolds, 1975).

Cognitive function may be defined as the ability of the brain to use information about and from the environment in which it lives in an adaptive way, and is usually measured in the laboratory by psychological tests. Behaviour is related to ability to manage interpersonal relationships, and is usually measured by standardized rating scales of psychopathology. Cognitive function and behaviour are intimately linked, but in our experimental paradigms we have chosen to consider them separately.

Table I   Incidence of side effects in a sample of 312 children with epilepsy

Side effect	No. of patients with side effects	Percentage
Distractability	31	9.9
Irritability	9	2.9
Slowing	60	19.2
Drowsiness	10	3.2
Depression	16	5.1
Fall in IQ > 15 points	32 (of 204 tested)	15.7
Neurotic disorder	82	26.3
Conduct	132	42.3

ANTICONVULSANT THERAPY AND FALL IN IQ

Our investigations began with the examination of epileptic children resident at a hospital school for children (Trimble and Corbett, 1980). A significant percentage of these children were noted to have undergone a deterioration of their intellectual quotient greater than 15 points on two intelligence tests separated by at least one year (Table I). These children had significantly higher serum levels of phenytoin and primidone than the rest of the population. This problem did not appear to be related to seizure frequency, the results being similar, particularly with regard to phenytoin, when children having only a small number of seizures were re-examined.

SERUM LEVELS AND BEHAVIOUR

In contrast, in that study it was more difficult to ascertain relationships between anticonvulsant prescription and behaviour disturbances; with regard to serum level assessments, only one significant difference emerged, namely that between carbamazepine and phenobarbitone. Carbamazepine had a negative correlation with conduct disorder (the higher serum level correlating with lower scores on conduct disorder), whereas for phenobarbitone the correlation was positive (Fig. 1). Of children receiving phenobarbitone, 50% were rated as having conduct disorder.

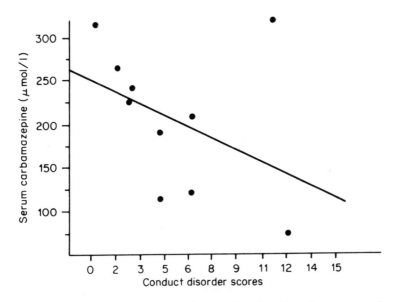

Fig. 1 Serum carbamazepine levels and disordered conduct – a negative correlation

TESTS FOR COGNITIVE FUNCTION

For assessing cognitive function, a test battery was designed at the National Hospitals; this was mainly free of practice effects, was of relevance to problems of cognitive function complained about by patients with epilepsy, and was thought to be sensitive to the effects of medication. In particular, memory, attention, concentration, mental speed and motor speed were assessed and patients were given subjective rating scales for the assessment of mood (Table II).

This battery was given to adult patients with epilepsy, and alteration of cognitive function in relation to changes of anticonvulsant therapy was assessed.

Table II Measures of cognitive function applied to population of adult patients with epilepsy (from Thompson and Trimble, 1982)

Function	Measure
Memory	
Pictures	Immediate recall
Words	Delayed recall
	Recognition
	Errors
Concentration	Visual scanning
	Auditory scanning
	Stroop test
Mental speed	Recognition threshold
	Pictures
	Words
Decision-making	Colour
	Category
	Visuo-motor response
Motor speed	Tapping
Mood	Subjective rating scales
	Mood adjective checklist
	Middlesex Hospital questionnaire

IMPROVED PERFORMANCE WITH DRUG REDUCTION OR CARBAMAZEPINE SUBSTITUTION

In the first studies, changes of performance on the test battery of three groups of patients were monitored. Medication changes were undertaken for two groups, the first consisting of 20 patients on polytherapy who had their treatment rationalized by reduction of the anticonvulsant load. The second group comprised 15 patients whose original medication had been withdrawn or reduced and who were prescribed carbamazepine, seven being changed to carbamazepine as monotherapy. The third group consisted of 10 patients who were kept on stable anticonvulsant therapy throughout and did not show marked fluctuations of serum anticonvulsant levels during the study: this group acted as controls. Patients were seen on three occasions, at three-monthly intervals, and medication was changed after the first session. At each session patients performed the neuropsychological tests and a blood sample was taken for analysis of serum drug levels.

The overall findings suggested that drug changes in both groups resulted in improvements in performance of the psychological tests and in mood. Comparable changes were not seen in the patients on stable therapy, and the findings did not appear to be the result of practice effects. In the first group,

Table III   Changes in test scores of patients undergoing drug reduction at the three three-monthly sessions

Functions and tests	Significance of differences between test scores at the three sessions (1, 2 and 3)
Psychological tests	
Mental speed	
Perceptual speed for words	1 vs 2; 1 vs 3***
Decision-making for colour	1 vs 3*
Decision-making for category	1 vs 3*
Motor speed	
Tapping rate: dominant hand	1 vs 2; 1 vs 3**
non-dominant hand	1 vs 2; 1 vs 3**
both hands	1 vs 2; 1 vs 3***
Attention	
Visual scanning: alone	1 vs 3; 2 vs 3*
with auditory task	1 vs 3; 2 vs 3*
total number scanned	1 vs 3*
total number of errors	1 vs 3*
Memory	
Pictures: delayed recall	1 vs 3*

*$P<0.05$; **$P<0.01$; ***$P<0.001$.

that undergoing a reduction of polypharmacy towards monotherapy, improvements were most marked in measures of concentration and motor speed and least marked in memory (Table III). Interestingly, these observed benefits were generally not seen until the third assessment session, namely, six months after drug changes. Improvements in mood, particularly anxiety and depression, were also noted. Patients changing to carbamazepine, either alone or in combination with existing medication, displayed more widespread improvements in test performance, particularly on measures of memory. These were generally apparent three months after a drug change and were maintained at the sixth-month session (Table IV). Moreover, in this group there was a trend towards improved seizure control across the sessions, significant in the case of tonic-clonic seizures.

SERUM ANTICONVULSANT LEVELS AND TEST SCORES

Two other studies explored the relationship between anticonvulsant serum levels and neuropsychological functioning. In these investigations, patients were seen on two occasions separated by an interval of three months. After the first session,

Table IV   Changes in test scores of patients undergoing drug reductions and carbamazepine substitution

Functions and tests	Significance of differences between test scores at the three sessions (1, 2 and 3)
Psychological tests	
Mental speed	
Perceptual speed for words	1 vs 2; 1 vs 3*
Perceptual speed for pictures	1 vs 2; 1 vs 3**
Decision-making for colour	1 vs 2; 1 vs 3**
Decision-making for category	1 vs 2; 1 vs 3**
Motor speed	
Tapping rate: dominant hand	1 vs 2; 1 vs 3**
non-dominant hand	1 vs 2; 1 vs 3**
both hands	1 vs 2; 1 vs 3***
Attention	
Visual scanning: alone	1 vs 2; 1 vs 3**
with auditory task	1 vs 2; 1 vs 3**
total number scanned	1 vs 2; 1 vs 3***
Memory	
Pictures: immediate recall	1 vs 2; 1 vs 3*
delayed recall	1 vs 2; 1 vs 3**
recognition	1 vs 3
Words: immediate recall	1 vs 2; 1 vs 3**
delayed recall	1 vs 2; 1 vs 3***

*$P < 0.05$; **$P < 0.01$; ***$P < 0.001$.

patients had their dosage changed in either direction; thus at one session patients had a higher serum level and at the other it was lower (Table V). In the first investigation on patients who were receiving polytherapy, the overall findings indicated that the mean scores for patients were lower on all but three measures

Table V   Mean serum levels of anticonvulsant (μmol/l) in the high-serum-level and low-serum-level sessions

Anticonvulsant	No. of patients	Session	
		High-serum level	Low-serum level
Phenytoin	6	53.2	32.5
Primidone	2	34.0	27.0
Carbamazepine	8	34.3	20.1
Sodium valproate	4	378.8	175.8

in the high-serum-level session in comparison with those in the low-serum-level session. This was statistically significant on six measures, including tests of concentration, mental speed and retention of new information.

In the last investigation, patients on monotherapy with phenytoin, carbamazepine and sodium valproate were examined on two occasions, at high and low concentrations, with an interval of three months between tests. Significant impairments in performance were observed when high- and low-serum level sessions were compared, being most marked for patients on phenytoin and sodium valproate. The impairments were mainly on tests of concentration and decisionmaking. In contrast, the carbamazepine-treated group showed only minimal differences between performances at high and low serum levels.

CONCLUSIONS

These studies, taken in conjunction with other work carried out in our laboratory, lead to the following conclusions with regard to anticonvulsant drugs, cognitive function and behaviour:

(a)   Phenytoin, in both patient and volunteer studies, impairs cognitive function across a wide spectrum of activity, and in some investigations the serum level relationship is such that increasing the levels leads to increased impairment

(b)   With sodium valproate and carbamazepine the impact on cognitive function is far less marked, although with sodium valproate a serum level relationship is seen

(c)   Carbamazepine appears to provoke minimal impairment of cognitive function, and improvement in performance has been indicated on some test results

(d)   The data on phenobarbitone are difficult to collect and the results to date are hard to interpret. However, this drug is generally thought to be sedative and to impair cognitive function.

In contrast to the data now accumulated on cognitive function, information on the relationship between anticonvulsants and behaviour disorder in epilepsy is difficult to interpret, although our own studies using standardized rating scales to assess mood show that rationalization of polytherapy improves symptoms of depression and anxiety. Of more significance in this respect is the growing literature on the use of carbamazepine in non-epileptic patients, recently reviewed in detail (Post et al., 1985), and also made the subject of a book (Emrich et al., 1984). Generally, carbamazepine has a mood-stabilizing effect similar to that of lithium, and is as effective as major tranquillizers in the control of acute mania. It may also be of value in the management of aggressive patients without epilepsy, and in some cases of schizophrenia. The results of these trials, where a confounding effect of the epilepsy does not have to be taken into account, seem to suggest psychotropic properties for carbamazepine.

REFERENCES

EMRICH, H. M., OKUMA, T., and MULLER, A. A. (1984) *Anticonvulsants in Affective Disorders*. Excerpta Medica, Amsterdam.

POST, R. M., UHDE, T. W., JOFFE, R. T., ROY-BYRNE, P. P., and KELLNER C. (1985) Anticonvulsants in psychiatric practice: New treatment – alternative and theoretical implications. In: *The Psychopharmacology of Epilepsy*, (1985) (Ed. M. R. Trimble). John Wiley and Sons, Chichester.

REYNOLDS, E. H. (1975) Chronic antiepileptic toxicity: a review. *Epilepsia*, **16**, 319–352.

THOMPSON, P., and TRIMBLE, M. R. (1982) Anticonvulsant drugs and cognitive functions. *Epilepsia*, **23**, 531–544.

TRIMBLE, M. R., and CORBETT, J. A. (1980) Behavioural and cognitive disturbances in epileptic children. *Ir. Med. J.*, **73** (Suppl. 10), 21–28.

Discussion

Dr E. H. Reynolds: Dr MacArdle described the very variable reported incidence of recurrent seizures after a single afebrile fit in childhood. Estimates for the risk in adults have also varied from 20 to 80%. I would like to offer an explanation for these diverse figures. Most of the published reports come from hospital clinics, where the patient is usually seen after a delay of at least several weeks and maybe several months. There is evidence that the sooner the patient is seen after a single fit, the higher will be the recorded rate of recurrence. The later he is seen, the lower the recurrence rate. In adult populations the overall risk of recurrence after a single fit is probably around 70 or 80%. This was implied by Gowers a century ago (Gowers, 1881), and has been confirmed both by a recent community study by Goodridge and Shorvon (1983) and in our own study with Dr Elwes (not yet published), which identified patients presenting to GPs and casualty officers. After an interval of three months, the overall risk of recurrence will have diminished by a third. This can be important in deciding when to initiate therapy.

Dr C. Rolles (Southampton): Dr MacArdle, you mentioned that anticonvulsants should be withdrawn slowly. How slowly? Is it possible that withdrawing drugs over six months simply extends the period of treatment, compared to withdrawal over six weeks?

MacArdle: The highest relapse rate occurs in the first few months after stopping treatment. The current MRC anticonvulsant withdrawal study is looking at a slow rate of withdrawal over a period of six months.

Reynolds: Dr MacArdle is right. Nobody knows the appropriate rate at which to withdraw medication, and this question has not been systematically investigated.

Dr R. S. Ackroyd (Cheltenham): In seeking to steer between adverse effects on cognitive function and giving a large enough dose to have the desired anticonvulsant effect, what level of drug dosage would you choose in a child who has had, say, two fits, been put on anticonvulsants, and then had no further fit? Should dosage be increased to keep pace with growth?

MacArdle: Our usual practice is to continue with the same dose, and not increase it as the child gets older unless there is a subsequent seizure.

Ackroyd: Would you not stop treatment sooner in that case, rather than go on for four years?

149

MacArdle: I do not think we have yet got a factual basis for deciding, but from the information we do have, the longer a child remains seizure free on treatment the better the long-term outlook. In practice, decisions tend to be made with the parents and the child, who will often be taken off treatment after two years.

Ackroyd: How often would you measure blood levels? And would you increase the dosage, say within the first year of starting, to reach a therapeutic level or be content with a lower level if the child was free of fits?

Reynolds: There are some misconceptions about what constitutes a therapeutic level. In adult populations, about one-third of our new referrals are controlled by low doses and low blood levels of the anticonvulsant drugs that we monitor. It is not necessary in all patients to push the dose up into the so-called therapeutic or optimum range. Using a small dose is fine if the fits remain controlled, but if fits recur you may have to push the dose into the optimum range. This is in line with Dr Trimble's evidence that it is best to keep patients on a low dose if possible.

Trimble: The serum levels of sodium valproate are not very helpful, because its half-life is so short, but some studies again suggest that seizures in some patients can be controlled on quite low doses.

Dr G. P. McMullin (Warrington): Since serum levels of anticonvulsants do not seem to be very relevant, might not cellular levels be more relevant, perhaps using red or white blood cells for the measurements?

Trimble: I do not know about blood cells, but Miss Coull, working with me, has been studying salivary levels in children; these are not proving very helpful in relation to dosage.

Ms C. Coull (London): Carbamazepine and phenytoin are difficult to measure. Most of the children have been on carbamazepine and I can really comment only on that. Carbamazepine levels tend to fluctuate widely during the day, but I do not know if that is just attributable to measuring saliva or whether it is due to fluctuation of blood levels throughout the day.

McMullin: I would like to suggest that somebody in a position to do cell studies might perhaps take them up.

Reynolds: Serum levels are extremely valuable in managing patients, to identify poor compliance and to keep the treatment simple by avoiding polytherapy. These are the most valuable aspects of monitoring and I am not sure that you would get better results by measuring drug levels in red or white cells or in the saliva.

Green: I would like to ask Dr Trimble if, in a child on monotherapy, when seizures are quite well controlled but there is some doubt about cognitive function, he would ever reduce the dose, even though it may not be above the therapeutic range, to try and improve cognitive function – at the risk of getting breakthrough seizures.

Trimble: The answer to this very important and practical question is that it depends on what the monotherapy is. A child on monotherapy with phenytoin I would change to valproate or carbamazepine. We do not think that children or adults on carbamazepine suffer much in the way of cognitive impairment. With sodium valproate, there is some evidence of dose-related cognitive impairment, so I would be prepared to lower the dose because it may be possible to do so without loss of control. Usually my worry would be monotherapy with phenytoin in a child with intellectual problems at school, cognitive deficits or memory function problems. I am not attributing every cognitive problem to that drug – a memory deficit, for example, can be related to seizure disturbance in the temporal lobe – but changing from phenytoin to carbamazepine or sodium valproate can bring with it marked improvements.

Dr A. J. Franklin (Chelmsford): Surely there is a lot of individual variation? I have certainly seen a case of impaired cognitive function on carbamazepine which did not appear with other drugs.

Trimble: Yes, of course you get idiosyncratic responses. We occasionally see an encephalopathy with sodium valproate and it has been well described. Drowsiness quite often occurs initially on carbamazepine, but it does not pose much of a problem.

Franklin: I mean rapid deterioration in work.

Trimble: I have not particularly seen that, but no drug is free from idiosyncratic responses, and they all deserve attention.

Franklin: Is there evidence of a blood–brain barrier with anticonvulsants? How do drug levels in the blood compare with brain concentrations?

Reynolds: There is variable penetration of the brain with all these drugs, but it has been shown quite conclusively in both animal and human studies that there is a very good correlation between the blood level, the serum level and the brain or CSF level. Although the serum levels quoted as therapeutic or optimal would not be exactly the same in the brain, the correlation is good enough for serum levels to be used in practice.

Trimble: Positron-emission tomography has shown that the epileptic focus takes up phenytoin as well as anywhere else in the brain, but this does not necessarily mean that seizures are controlled.

Franklin: Suppose you have a boy of 15½ who has had a first fit, without recurrence, and asks if he can apply for a driving licence, what would you say?

Verity: The question now on the application form has been made very much more specific. Applicants have to be free of seizures at least during the day, on or off therapy, for two years before being allowed a driving licence. So it would be no use for your boy to apply.

Eeg-Olofsson: Could Mike Trimble tell us the time of day when plasma levels are measured in relation to disturbances in cognitive function and behaviour? I ask because there is a tremendous fluctuation in plasma levels during the 24 hours. In a study on the saliva concentration of carbamazepine in 40 children, we found that many of them had a quite normal level in the morning before taking the dose of Tegretol. But after three hours many of them had high levels, above the therapeutic range. Those children sometimes showed tiredness, which could be considerable, and we had to lower the dose and, in some cases, change to three doses a day. With lower levels over the day, the children became better.

Trimble: In these studies the serum or salivary levels are taken immediately after the testing period, because we are trying to relate the changes in psychological tests to the serum concentration.

Aicardi: The problem of drug levels is becoming more complicated now that we have the slow-release forms of valproate, for example. You never know at what time the peak or trough level of the drug will occur. This depends very much upon individual factors, such as what you have eaten the day before. I am not sure whether it applies to carbamazepine. Everything depends on what you want to show. If a child is suspected of being intoxicated, then you would sample at the time of maximum effect. If the problem was a breakthrough seizure you would obtain the fasting level.

Reynolds: Dr Verity presented some very important prospective data from community studies and concluded that the prognosis for most children with epilepsy is very good – although much of the literature from specialized centres suggests the opposite. In following adolescents and adults who presented to us with previously untreated epilepsy for the first time, we have found that most do well on treatment, with something like 75% going into remission. It is becoming clear that the prognosis for most patients with epilepsy is good, although much of the literature from specialized centres suggests the opposite.

Corbett: One of the interesting points from the National Development Studies is the remarkable consistency in prevalence rates over the years since 1946. Why should this be so?

Verity: Another surprising thing is the lack of association between perinatal problems and subsequent febrile *and* afebrile seizures.

Green: I wonder how much we know about the management of children with a first afebrile seizure who are otherwise well. It may be that we are seeing an even more biased sample than we think if some are not reported to the GP and others are not referred to a paediatrician unless they have further seizures. If so, the results for one or two seizures could be very much better than these studies show.

Verity: Yes. In the NCDS, 45% were admitted to hospital, and 65% in the Child Health and Education Study. In other words, despite the fact that febrile seizures can be such terrifying things, many of these children do not seem to get referred to hospital and some have not even seen the doctor – although the mother may later describe what sounds very much like a febrile convulsion. With afebrile seizures, in children or later in life, there are all sorts of social pressures not to admit that these things have occurred, and presumably there is quite a percentage of such unrecognized cases in the community at large.

Aicardi: What is the incidence in this type of study of possibly misdiagnosing something which is not epileptic as epilepsy? The inclusion of a significant proportion of such cases could certainly affect the figures.

Verity: I do not think it is possible to answer that question on the basis of this type of study. Even when Gastaut reviewed his own data on patients who had been seen by him or his staff he was unable to come to a final conclusion about the diagnosis in quite a large percentage of patients; obviously the studies I discussed are nowhere near as closely involved with the patients.

REFERENCES

GOODRIDGE, D. G. M., and SHORVON, S. D. (1983) Epileptic seizures in a population of 6000. II. Treatment and prognosis. *Br. Med. J.*, **287**, 645–647.
GOWERS, W. R. (1881) *Epilepsy and Other Chronic Convulsive Disorders: Their Causes, Symptoms and Treatment.* Churchill, London.

Panel discussion

Dr Euan Ross, Dr Brian Bower, Dr Keith Brown, Professor
Niall O'Donohoe, Dr Edward Reynolds

Dr M. I. Maguire (Merthyr Tydfil): How long should one continue with prophylactic
anticonvulsants after neonatal convulsions due to asphyxia? We are treating asphyxiated
newborns vigorously with anticonvulsants at the beginning, but it is hard to judge when
they can safely be stopped.

Brown: Tonic fits within the first 24 hours, following asphyxia, carry quite a marked
risk of long-term seizure problems. By 48 hours the seizures are nearly always clonic
or hemiclonic, and these have no significance at all for long-term prognosis. They are
more likely to be due to secondary metabolic complications than asphyxia. If a neonate
is still having fits 10–14 days after birth, then they are not due to perinatal problems
but to cortical dysplasia or some other abnormality.

We used to keep babies with post-asphyxial tonic fits in the first 24 hours on medication
for four weeks and then tail it off. However, one of the problems is that if you are giving
high-dose barbiturate therapy, withdrawal may provoke seizures. After prolonged high
dosage we therefore start to withdraw at two to three months. After conventional short-
term therapy at lower dosage, we start tailing off by three to four weeks. If the child
convulses after the first three or four weeks of life, then he may well go on to partial
seizures or infantile spasms.

I believe we should treat epilepsies as arrhythmias of the nervous system – *acute*
or *chronic*. An acute arrhythmia with an acute asphyxial episode or acute meningitis
or an acute encephalitic illness ought to be treated for a limited period as an acute
complication of an acute disease. Only with a chronic arrhythmia is long-term therapy
needed.

Ross: Barbiturate therapy has probably had its longest reign in neonatal seizures. Is
it still going to be the drug of choice in years to come?

Brown: Barbiturates are being given for different reasons now, not so much to control
seizures but for cerebral protection against focal ischaemia. The evidence of protection
against global ischaemia is not so good; it is very difficult to show that high-dose
barbiturates reduce cerebral oedema and thus decrease intracranial pressure, thereby giving

cerebral protection. In an older child, monitoring of intracranial pressure coupled with cranial signs means that you can give thiopentone in appropriate dosage to lower the intracranial pressure, and then change to pentobarbitone for maintenance. But in the neonate the benefits of high-dose barbiturates are uncertain; in terms of cerebral protection, you have no guide to dosage – which means that you have to settle for the upper end of the therapeutic range.

By contrast, the benefits of phenobarbitone for neonatal seizures are becoming clearer. In our own experience, neonates with a seizure following asphyxia 10 years ago had long-term morbidity of 46%. Nowadays, with intensive treatment of neonatal seizures, the long-term morbidity is 12%. In other words, a full-term baby with a seizure following intrapartum asphyxia that is vigorously treated now carries less than one-third the morbidity risk, compared with 10 years ago.

Dr B. D. Bower (Oxford): Why not treat for about 10 days following an asphyxial convulsion, as we do, and then stop the barbiturate – or whatever anticonvulsant is used – to see whether seizures recur? In the majority they won't. The objection to continuing with barbiturate is, of course, the anxiety we all have about its possible effects on the immature developing brain.

Eeg-Olofsson: I agree completely with Dr Brown, but would like to add one thing, which is in line with Dr Bower's comment. The EEG is very useful in the neonatal period – to settle the prognosis and show whether to stop anticonvulsant therapy or not. If the EEG is normal, you can safely drop the therapy after about 10 days or so. But if the EEG shows pathological bursts, you have to continue therapy, even if the child has no seizures. I treat these children with phenobarbitone for no more than one month; if treatment is still needed after that, I use carbamazepine or valproate.

O'Donohoe: Perhaps the original questioner was thinking of an analogy with head injury – which has sometimes been used to justify long-term treatment in newborns who had seizures. The idea is to inhibit kindling, but since long-term anticonvulsant therapy has not been shown to prevent later epilepsy after head injury, it probably is not valid in babies either.

Ross: Kindling is an extremely important debating issue for paediatricians. We need to make up our minds whether the phenomenon really exists in children as distinct from laboratory animals. If so, do some children kindle more easily than others?

O'Donohoe: Relatively incombustible material, as Lennox said, requires a blazing torch to set it alight – a severe insult or perhaps a convulsant drug – whereas genetically combustible material may light much more easily. That is the point I was trying to make about the interaction between epileptogenicity on the one hand and acquired injury or abnormality on the other. Dr Aicardi and others have stressed the importance of childhood infection in the first few years of life – not febrile convulsions – in causing minor brain injury.

Aicardi: Yes, I think this still has some importance but probably less than it used to have at this age because general improvement in the care of young children has included better care of infections. Nonetheless I have no doubt that quite a number of childhood epilepsies are due to the sequelae of brain infections.

Green: We do not want to start therapy in children who may not have epilepsy, after a single seizure, for example, but are there situations in which we should not treat established epilepsy? Some people would not treat benign rolandic epilepsy or occasional petit mal or some nocturnal seizures, but Robinson (1984) has recently argued that all these ought to be treated because of the kindling effect.

Reynolds: Among adults and adolescents, I would not treat alcoholics who presented with seizures or people who, for one reason or other, I was firmly convinced would not comply with therapy. Many factors have to be weighed up when making the decision whether or not to treat children or adults who present with one or more fits. I place a great deal of weight on the views of the patient and relatives, their personalities and whether or not they seem likely to comply with treatment. But, having said that, I am also concerned that fits can beget more fits. If they are allowed to get out of control, there is a risk that control may be difficult or impossible to establish. Certainly our own evidence suggests that, in new referrals treated with a single anticonvulsant, if the fits are not controlled within the first year or two, it is unlikely that they ever will be. Our inclination is to try to get on top of epilepsy as rapidly as possible, in an attempt to get the best possible prognosis. In short, there are arguments for going in hard and fast with treatment in many cases, and there are other arguments for holding off in certain situations.

Corbett: We are committing some children to very long-term anticonvulsant treatment while their brains are developing. We do know that, for example, phenytoin depresses folate levels, which are important in neurotransmission and might, therefore, affect brain development. But what do we actually know about the long-term effects of anticonvulsants on cognition and behaviour in man or animals? Most studies seem to have been short term.

Reynolds: This is research which should be but to my knowledge has not yet been done.

Trimble: So far as I know we have no long-term studies of the effects of anticonvulsant drugs on brain maturation. Folic acid does, however, appear to be a very important variable, low levels being significantly associated with psychiatric and cognitive disturbances in patients with epilepsy.

Reynolds: Several studies of folate deficiency have shown a relationship not only to epilepsy but also to a wide range of neuropsychiatric disorders, especially depression and dementia. It is a very complicated subject. A recent community study in the King's area has shown the usual high incidence of drug-induced folate deficiency in epileptic patients and a very close association between drug-induced folate deficiency and depression. This is not a dietary folate deficiency as a result of depression, but drug-induced deficiency that may be playing some causative role in the depression.

Dr G. P. McMullin (Warrington): Dr Verity showed one slide indicating a significant relationship between febrile convulsions and hearing and speech defects. That might tie up with the possible importance of frequent infection in young children. Secondly, I wonder if the distinction between febrile and afebrile convulsion is always satisfactory. Suppose a child has a cold or minor infection, but does not develop much in the way of a fever, and then develops a convulsion, how should it be classified?

O'Donohoe: With regard to the treatment or non-treatment of epilepsy with drugs, I should like to stress the importance of benign centro-temporal rolandic epilepsy. It really is extremely common, accounting for about one in every five childhood epilepsies. If you treat them initially, they may only ever have one seizure. If you put them on drugs, you may never know whether they would have had another. Children with this extraordinary condition certainly do remarkably well; even those who do not improve at first eventually progress to 100% remission. The prognosis is very good, and this is probably an argument against routine drug treatment, despite what I have said about kindling.

Bower: In my practice, there is growing reluctance on the part of parents to treating a child with drugs. Some 'don't believe' in them, while others wrap it up in more sophisticated language, but the onus is coming on us as doctors to prove that anticonvulsant therapy is in fact necessary in certain instances.

Ross: This has been an excellent meeting. There is much to be gained from relaxed but academic discussion on the needs of children with epilepsy – from provision of services and treatment to fundamental research. We are grateful to Ciba-Geigy for hosting the meeting and hope that they would like to do this again because there is so much more thinking to be done about children's epilepsies and scope for new research initiatives.

I should also thank you all for coming and being very lively discussants. Then I must give our very special thanks to the many speakers, particularly to Professor Jean Aicardi from France and Professor Eeg-Olofsson from Sweden, for contributing so much to the success of the meeting.

REFERENCE

ROBINSON, R. J. (1984) When to start and stop anticonvulsants. In: *Recent Advances in Paediatrics*, 7, pp. 155–174 (Ed. R. Meadow). Churchill Livingstone, Edinburgh.

Index